This Girl Can (Sometimes)

Maria 慧 Claridge

Copyright © 2021 Maria 慧 Claridge

All rights reserved.

ISBN-13: 979-8-5995-4575-0

THIS GIRL CAN (SOMETIMES)

DEDICATION

I dedicate this book to all readers struggling with mental health issues.

ACKNOWLEDGMENTS

I would like to give special thanks to my dearest friend Alistair.

I would also like to thank my partner Daisuke for all his love and support.

I would like to thank my book editor and wonderful friend, Lexi Dutnall.

THIS GIRL CAN (SOMETIMES)

INTRODUCTION

This Girl Can (Sometimes)

Blind-sided by a black cloud falling upon me,
Swallowing me whole, it gives no mercy.
If only there was something you could take
To make it stop – to give that quick escape.
Finding the strength to reach out can be hard;
Desperate to breathe, I don't want to be scarred.
I know there's someone who hears my calls
To grant me inner peace and end my falls.
It's fine if today you just managed to survive,
Now take a deep breath, pause and revive.

THIS GIRL CAN (SOMETIMES)

PROLOGUE

I feel exposed and vulnerable.

I want mental health to be spoken about, and I want to remove all negative stigma surrounding it. I never thought I would be writing a book about mental health, but then again, I never planned to be mentally ill. It is daunting to think that in this book, I will be revealing my condition and darkest moments to all my family, friends and work clients. But I want people to know that you can have any mental health illness and still have a fulfilling life full of love and light.

Through this book, I want to share what has worked for me, what hasn't worked for me, and how I became okay with having mental health issues for life. This is not to suggest that what worked for me will work for you, but know you are not alone in your journey.

I have gone through loves and breakups, friendships and abandonments, moments of courage as well as moments of vulnerability.

I have worked on myself and will continue to do so from here on out.

I invite you to read this book with both an open mind and an open heart.

THIS GIRL CAN (SOMETIMES)

CHAPTER 1

I think about suicide every so often. I blame it on having bipolar, but sometimes I just don't feel worthy enough to be alive.

I have a home, shelter and food. I have a lovely supportive family, a partner who really loves me, I enjoy my work and have fun and loving friends…yet sometimes I feel empty.

There are days I perform, smiling and laughing, going through the motions of living, but inside I feel a part of me dying.

In my dark times, if I were able to, I would slit my wrists open and simply be done with it all. But I'm not able to. I don't like inflicting pain on myself. I gave myself a hard slap across the face once and decided self-infliction wasn't for me, and I would never do it again.

I know what to do and do all the things to keep myself healthy. I eat well. I exercise. I practice yoga and meditate in the morning. I keep my days structured. I am content working for myself. I set small goals and I work hard. I have lovely clients and people in my life, and on good days I feel I have purpose and I'm making a small difference in the world.

But this emptiness…it comes in many forms.

There are days where I can't stop crying. There are evenings full of darkness. My counsellor or Lexi, my best friend, would tell me to 'embrace the tears and lean into the darkness.' But embracing this feeling can be so overwhelming. I feel like my head could explode.

All I know is that I can do this. I can ride out the storm.

This girl can. Well, sometimes.

Let us start at the beginning.

CHAPTER 2

Privilege and race

First of all, I cannot tell my story without talking about race. They are intrinsically linked. How I position myself and how other people perceive me is shaped, and continues to be shaped, by the events that have occurred throughout my life. The history of the world matters, and the privilege and discrimination I have experienced are woven into my story.

I am white, mixed race. My mum, Midori, is Japanese, and my dad, John, is English. Growing up in my hometown on the South Coast of England felt challenging at times with its lack of diversity. I encountered bullying, children tugging their eyes back in jest, and was often mistaken as being Chinese instead of Japanese. For a long time, a man at the Saturday market thought my mum ran the Chinese takeaway shop. This is how small-minded some of the town people were, and although tough, it made me realise how important it is to be inclusive and racially aware. As I grew older and more confident, I embraced my Japanese blood. Living in London, I met so many people from all walks of life.

I have had the privilege of being educated, going to university, travelling, access to health care and having a comfortable life. Not everyone has had these opportunities, and it saddens me to think that there are people in our world being judged by their race. There are also many people of colour who don't have the opportunity or access to the resources needed to address their mental health needs. Many do not have the space to talk through their issues and are being targeted or bullied, worsening their mental health. This is not okay.

I am very lucky to have had the opportunities that I did when it came to getting medical help for my mental health. I want to make clear that there are people out there with mental health issues who might not have the chance to share their experiences with the world because of their colour or background. I want to help change this.

Now, more than ever, it is important to have that chat with your friends about race and the importance of talking about one's mental health.

CHAPTER 3

Wait, what? Your mum doesn't run the Chinese takeaway?

LYMINGTON – THE TOWN IN ITS OWN BUBBLE

I grew up in a town called Lymington on the South Coast of England. It's one of those lovely, quaint seaside towns which is also close to the forest. My flatmate, Ingrid, once said, 'Lymington is the destination where birds have a vacation for the summer.' In the cold winter months, my friends and I take long forest walks or go around the Sea Wall, stopping for a coffee or hot chocolate at one of the local coffee shops. In the evenings, we go to the pubs, sit near a welcoming roaring fire in the corner, and drink ales or wine. In the summer, we spend much time out on the water in sailing boats or ribs, travelling to beaches around the Needles on the Isle of Wight. Walking the streets in the evening, you can look up and see the beautiful starlit night sky. I feel safe. So many amazing and fun magical moments happen in this small town.

My family home is near some beautiful gardens which have tennis courts, flower beds, a football and rugby pitch which are welcome for use by anyone. The space is vast, and the air fresh. I can sometime forget how lucky I was, to grow up in a loving home with endless outdoor adventures on my front doorstep.

Lymington is extremely quiet in comparison to the hustle and bustle of Tokyo, and I knew my mum struggled with making friends and fitting in when she first moved there. She occasionally encountered small-minded people, assuming she was Chinese and unable to speak any English. Speaking slowly and loudly to her, occasionally using gestures, it could be perceived comical. Despite English not being her first language and having a completely different upbringing in the heart of Japan, over her time in Lymington, she adapted. My mum created a new, beautiful life full of friendships and laughter.

My parents met through dinghy sailing. Both are keen sailors. My dad has a good reputation working as the local boat builder and is well-liked in Lymington. Both my parents work hard; dad works long hours at the boatyard, while mum manages all the finances.

My mum is beautiful and has a laugh so loud it is heard from any room in the house. Like me, her sense of humour is childlike (simple), and making her laugh makes me feel golden. Whilst I was growing up, she had long ink-black hair which framed her round face. Her petite Japanese build contradicts her fiery personality. If she was annoyed or mad you would soon know, but fortunately, once her wrath was out in the open, she would cool down quickly. My brother once slammed his bedroom door post-fight with mum, and mum responded with, 'I can slam my door, too!' before she slammed her own bedroom door. Dad wasn't impressed with the crack it caused in the downstairs ceiling.

My mum is the strongest person I know, and we have a very close relationship. This became abundantly clear to me for the first time, whilst we were travelling together in Sri Lanka. A woman exclaimed that she could never travel with her mum and get on as well as we did, making the observation my mum and I had a unique relationship. An observation I had never myself made until that moment.

My mum is open-minded about a lot of things, and as I grew older, we started talking more like friends do. Well, most of the time. She's still a mum.

My dad, with his thick builder hands, is tall and handsome. He now has silver hair, but still a defined jaw, with eyes radiating warmth and kindness. He is always thoughtful and never one to react with anger. I can only recall a handful of times he has ever raised his voice. He listens intently and pauses before speaking. Whenever I have been upset, he has come quietly into my room and sat on my bed, waiting until I was ready to speak.

If ever I'm in any trouble, I can always turn to mum or dad. I know all the good traits I have can be attributed to the two of them.

My parents make a beautiful pairing, and to this day, dad still comes home with flowers (reduced-priced, but still) and has mum laughing her sunny laugh. I love looking at photos of them together. Photos like the one of dad with his bushy moustache and flared trousers, pushing my brother in a buggy, our then-dog Shelly trotting alongside him, mum in her dungaree denim dress, belly swollen with me, holding dad's hand.

PRIVILEGED

Growing up, my parents provided my brother and I with a variety of opportunities. We were fortunate to be able to travel. We always took a family summer holiday. One summer, when I was 9, we went to Greece, where I fell in love with Greek yoghurt and honey, playing in the sunshine every day. From when we were babies, at Christmas time, we would travel to Japan. I can still picture Rob, my brother, at age 6, sprawled on two airplane chairs, me sprawled on the floor by the feet. This became harder to do as we grew older and bigger.

I struggled with maths at school, so I had math tutoring every Wednesday with Mr Lewis, whilst my brother attended private school - I didn't get the grades to go to private school. We both had piano lessons, and my parents endured me playing My Heart Will Go On from Titanic for three years.

During our school years, we attended gymnastic club after school and tennis club in the summer. I played volleyball and was part of the athletics club. We were both keen sailors and competed around the UK and internationally. The opportunities we had felt endless. To this day, I feel like an all-round athlete because we tried so many sports when we were younger.

Warm memories and gratitude spread through me when I think back over my childhood.

If I have children, I wish for them to have these same opportunities. I strongly believe trying a variety of things, experiencing different cultures, and all these sports and travel helped me build the character and healthy lifestyle I have today.

SCHOOL

My brother and I were the only two half-Asian children at our primary school. It was a small school, and on my very first day, I was excited to make new friends. My brother, on the other hand, was in floods of tears clinging onto mum. I feel this reflects how free and confident I was from a young age. I felt fearless, and this feeling I still recall and hold close. Although I did struggle in my early years, being the youngest in my year and falling asleep in class, I was a happy child and an average grade student. My brother excelled in all his subjects, to the point where sometimes he would even correct the teacher. Yet, despite the difference in academia and sailing ability, my parents never made me feel I needed to compete or prove my worth.

I enjoyed primary school and liked my friends, but this abruptly changed one day in the bathroom when my friends pointed out how small my eyes were in comparison to theirs. This triggered the beginning of my complex with my eyes. Some other children started chanting, 'Chinese, Chinese,' during break time. After a stern word from the teacher, the children apologised the next day, and things seemed okay again.

Upon reflection, I definitely noticed microaggressions and racism growing up. It was in the kinds of things that children would say out of curiosity with no ill intentions, but it still made me feel different.

According to Google, microaggression is 'a term used for verbal, behavioural, or environmental indignities, whether intentional or unintentional, that communicate hostile, derogatory, or negative prejudicial slights and insults toward any group, particularly culturally marginalised groups.'

Racism is a 'prejudice, discrimination, or antagonism directed against a person or people on the basis of their membership of a particular racial or ethnic group, typically one that is a minority or marginalized.'

What I experienced growing up wasn't right or healthy for a child to experience. If I ate my lunch with chopsticks, ate rice balls, onigiri, or did anything slightly Japanese, they'd say, 'Oh my god, you're weird,' or, 'Oh, it's because you're Asian.' These kinds of comments can be damaging, especially whilst growing up, strengthening the feeling of exclusion. When you're young, you want to fit in and feel 'normal'. Being told you are different by your peers builds barriers and insecurities.

I felt upset for being singled out, but forgiveness came easy to me as a child. I received the kindness award in my final year of Primary School, which my parents found heart-warming, and with my peers clapping, I felt I had finally been accepted.

BIG SCHOOL

Entering secondary school, my sense of acceptance, friendship, security and confidence within myself changed. Once again, I felt like an outsider. Again, lacking diversity, there was one other Asian boy in the year above me, and people instantly assumed we were related.

Age 12, I'm sitting on the bench with my friend, drinking our Capri Sun juices. She turns to me asking,

'Hey, your brother Freddie is in the year above us...'

'He's not my brother,' I cut in, squeezing my juice box, my body language cold. 'He's Chinese.'

'Yeh, yeh, same as you, though? Chinese and Japanese...they are pretty much the same, right?' she says knowingly, eyes narrowed, looking at me like I was behaving dim.

Anger pulses through my body. I want to scream at her that this is not the same. We aren't the same.

'Sure,' I flash a smile. 'Let's get to class.' What my friend didn't see was that my knuckles had turned white, and the juice box had buckled under the pressure of my clenched fist. Anything to avoid conflict. Standing up for myself was something I lacked at school, and that assertiveness I still sometimes lack now.

Differentiating between Asians can be difficult, but I feel one should never assume. Children should be educated that there are all kinds of cultures and ethnicities. If one thinks it's just children who make these assumptions, adults often think my Japanese, half-Filipino partner Dice and I are related. At parties, at the tennis club, etc., we often get asked if we are siblings. This is something which would never be assumed in London, only in this small town.

At secondary school, there were many times I wished I was white and had Western eyes. I would go to sleep at night thinking if I had Western eyes I wouldn't be picked on. I wouldn't be stereotyped. I thought boys would notice me more if I looked like my blonde and pretty friends. I became the poster diversity girl in the school catalogue and on the school reception wall, which resulted in me feeling like I was singled out as different from my peers. Growing up, there were definitely times I wished I wasn't Japanese.

I remember when my then best friend and some other kids started saying this rhyme which went 'Chinese, Japanese, Siamese,' and then they'd tug their eyes back. It made me feel ashamed of my eyes all over again. When choosing a Disney princess in games, I was always asked to be Mulan, even though I wanted to be the Little Mermaid, Ariel, as I loved the sea. But that didn't matter as Mulan has narrow eyes like me. I got called 'Jackie Chan' and nicknamed 'Chinky', and these words cut a wound so deep I cried myself to sleep at night. It was hurtful. I am not Chinese, and I despised being singled out for the shape of my eyes.

I remember on one occasion, I had tied my hair back into a new style and felt very pleased with the result, not being very good with hair or makeup. But when a group of boys walked past me and yelled, 'Nice hair, Jackie Chan,' I rushed to the closest bathroom, looked under the doors to check no one else was there, avoiding the mirrors, and shut myself in a cubicle. I put the toilet seat down and pulled my legs up, hugged them close and began sobbing. Pulling my hair down, and feeling the humiliation burn through me, fat tears rolled down my face. I would cry in the school bathrooms on a regular basis but always arrived home with a smile on my face, not wanting my parents to worry. But the damage had been done, their hurtful words had pierced my heart, and I no longer wished to be Japanese. It's sad to think my past self would denounce being Japanese for the sake of fitting in, but what child doesn't compare themselves to their classmates?

From then on, I would never tell my friends about going to Japan over Christmas, and I would go out of my way to hide anything I did or ate related to Japanese culture. I was ashamed of my Japanese heritage. It made me feel different, and like I didn't belong or fit in with my peers. They made me feel like it wasn't okay to be Japanese. So, sometimes, I behaved as a false extrovert to compensate for my lack of confidence.

UNIVERSITY – LONDON

When I moved to London for university, my whole world was turned upside down. Walking around London, I was surrounded by a fusion of different people, ages, life experiences and cultures. My peers were no longer a sea of white faces. There were other people who had grown up with two cultures or had been exposed to other cultures, and I began to flourish. I no longer needed to hide my Japanese heritage. I no longer felt singled out. In Lymington, without realising it, I had been holding my breath for all those years, and London gave me the space to finally breathe.

I sometimes wonder what it would have been like if I wasn't the only Asian girl in my year, or if we weren't the only Asian family in town. I wonder what it would have been like to have a city upbringing. But looking back, I definitely see value in the way I was raised in the open space and fresh air. I'm really grateful to have grown up between two cultures. I think my mum and dad raised me the best way they could, and upon reflection, I feel I have the best of both worlds.

Experiencing bullying during my school years allowed me to develop empathy and kindness for others. I never turned into someone who retaliated or became a bully.

Writing this, I realised more than ever how important it is for children to feel love and connection in order to grow and thrive. Children need to feel accepted when they are young, it's what morphs them into healthy adults. Love, security and acceptance were at the heart of my family life. But what happened at school was outside of their control.

My parents made it clear their love didn't depend on my accomplishments. None of my mistakes were treated like life failures. Children can feel fear and anxiety from experiences they don't understand, but my parents made my brother and I feel okay to be afraid or anxious. It's okay to be afraid of something at any point in your life.

Confidence grows in a home that is full of unconditional love and affection. We learn from our family how to form relationships and function in society and in our work. My parents are a team who support me, believe in me and care about me. If I didn't have their love and support whilst enduring the bullying, I would have felt isolated. Instead, I have many happy memories from my childhood and I showed no signs of depression or manic behaviour. I want to state very clearly that my parents could have never prevented what was going to happen to me in my early twenties when signs of mental health struggles started to materialise for me.

I call this time in my life, pre-bipolar diagnosis (PBD).

THIS GIRL CAN (SOMETIMES)

CHAPTER 4

"I had a dream, I got everything I wanted...they called me weak, like I'm not just somebody's daughter..." - Billie Eilish

My dream for my past self and future children: You walk into school and greet friends who have backgrounds from across the globe. You talk about different cultures, present interesting items that are sentimental to you. You learn each other's languages. There's no fear in being different. You each embrace your uniqueness. Every morning, you look in the mirror with pride. Everyone's eyes are different, everyone's skin colour is different. There's no pain in your eyes. Just love and acceptance. There are textbooks, picture books, media and films you see yourself in. You could be the lead, not just the karate master or a fun action sidekick.

I have hope.

THIS GIRL CAN (SOMETIMES)

CHAPTER 5

Fun Me vs. Depressed Me

JAKE

Jake, my boyfriend at the time, and I had another argument. He slammed the door behind him, and I knew his next destination would be his mum's. In my small London two-bedroom flat, I was glad my tenant was away. The walls were thin. Jake was very much a mummy's boy, and the slightest of conflicts would send him running home.

I called Tim sobbing. 'I will be there in 15,' he said. Tim put the phone down.

My flat is located between Greenwich and North Greenwich. I now call Lymington home, but my parents still have this London flat. Greenwich itself is beautiful, with the Cutty Sark and rolling green grounds. I liked living in Greenwich as it didn't feel like London. It had a similar small-town feel to Lymington. My flat had a Japanese vibe, low table, floor seat and Japanese art decor. Jake had always felt the space was very much mine, and he was right.

I was 25, and living with Jake had seemed like a great idea at the time. The relationship had escalated quickly.

On our second date, we went clubbing in central London. A few drinks in, my body moving to the beat of the music, wearing a red, figure-hugging dress, I opened my eyes to see his blue eyes staring back at me. He leaned in, and, bodies now touching, my hands ran down his strong arms. I threw my head back, smiling. I fancied Jake. I wanted a bit of fun, and it started off as just that, but I needed to be needed. I needed to be desired. I depended on external validation, and Jake gave it to me. I asked him to move in a few weeks after.

A fitness couple, I thought we were in love. He was blond, built and adorable, like a Labrador. I admit now, our conversations never had much depth, but we always had fun. Our relationship was mostly based on clubbing, Instagram pictures and gyming. He was a funny guy and often had me falling over laughing. We lived very much in the moment, and we were a very Instagramable couple.

I learnt it is never sustainable to be a couple constantly living in the moment. Inevitably, the past needs to be explored - things can resurface, and the future needs some thinking about to ensure your paths, values and goals align.

I began investing more in Jake, helping him with his finances, savings, and supported him in all his interests. Anything he needed; I was there. I enjoyed spending time with his family, and every Sunday, we would travel to his family home in Greenwich to have a roast dinner. I grew close to his family, often looking after his younger brother or walking the dogs. At the time, it made sense for him to move in. I thought we were building a future. My mum had warned me Jake was a 'Fun boy' and felt uneasy about our future. I don't think my brother liked Jake. When he came to Lymington to stay, my brother didn't make eye contact or attempt any engagement in conversation. The dinner table felt chilly.

'Your brother is rude,' Jake folded his arms, sitting down on my bed.

'Mmm, no. He just doesn't feel the need to always speak. Give him some time, he will warm up to you.' The lie burned my lips.

After Jake left the flat, I was angry. Collapsing on the sofa, I sighed, burying my face in my palms. Deep down, I knew this wasn't all his fault. I knew I was feeling depressed, and this was taking a toll on us. My relationship with food was becoming destructive again. I had struggled with eating disorders before, but this was the first time Jake had seen this side of me. I had slowly gained weight over the months. Work had been slow, I was not being proactive, and I was feeling vulnerable. Jake had met me in my prime, when I was in the gym daily, setting up my PR company and had a fun, social life.

'Fun me', I thought.

Jake fell in love with 'Fun me'. I think back to when we were playing around with Acro Yoga in Greenwich Park. He had taken a snap of me mid-laugh, looking at him adoringly. He wanted nothing to do with the 'Depressed me', slumped, binging junk food on the sofa.

What's happened to me? How have I let things slip this badly?

There was a knock on the door. I got up from the sofa, walked down the corridor and opened the heavy door to find Tim. He was wearing his leather jacket, jeans, and his Timberland boots. Tim, built like a machine, has brains as well as the ability to connect with people. Macho as ever, he came in and bundled me into his arms. We went into the living room. He took his place on the sofa as I moved to the Japanese-style floor chair.

I clapped my hands together. 'Jake wants to break up.' My voice was surprisingly chipper.

Staring deep into my eyes, Tim said nothing. There was a glint in his knowing green eyes.

'I think we probably should break up. He's just not understanding why I am so down.' Tim nodded his head, listening intently. Tim was always a great listener.

'It sounds like you are okay with breaking up?'

THIS GIRL CAN (SOMETIMES)

'I am!' The epiphany struck as I realised how I perked up to answer his question. I paused before asking, 'Tim, stay the night?'

'Yes.'

Tim knew I struggled with sleep, and I didn't want to be alone. It was late. 'Let's get ready for bed,' Tim said, standing up.

I looked at Tim as he slept. Good friends now, but half a year ago, Tim had asked me out on a date. I wear a chain with a pendant that spells my name in Egyptian hieroglyphics. It had been a gift from my Egyptian friends when I had travelled there with my mum. Tim had boldly come up to me in the gym and had read the pendant. 'So, you must be Maria?' He had smiled warmly. Since then, we'd been chatty in the gym, and after one session, he dramatically slammed his free weights down and marched over to where I was sitting. 'Maria, will you go out with me?' He was so vulnerable at that moment, I was speechless. It was very sweet, but I had just met Jake and I was besotted. However, I could never quite let Tim go. He was a stable friend and gave me a sense of security. I needed him in my life, always.

My phone lit up on the bedside table. It was Jake. 'I'm outside.' I quickly pulled on a hoodie and some trackies and tiptoed out of the room, not wanting to make any noise to wake Tim. I closed the bedroom door behind me. I walked down the concrete stairs to the ground floor. I knew Jake would be furious if he knew Tim was at the flat, let alone in our bed. I faced Jake outside the building.

'Jake, it's late.'

'Babe, I'm sorry. I love you. You know I do.'

'Jake...'

Those three words, I love you, can be so powerful. When you say a true 'I love you' to a person, you are being brave and vulnerable. A true 'I love you' can change your whole world as

I would discover later. When there is love in your life, everything seems much brighter and more beautiful. I wanted Jake's love, I wanted to feel secure, and I believed his love would be the solution to many of my problems. My reality would be illuminated in a way that only Jake's love could provide. But Jake didn't love me. He, too, had a fear of being alone.

True romantic love can be one of the most transformational and supportive experiences. I realise now this 'I love you' from Jake came from empty lips. But in that moment, I could feel myself wondering if we could work things out. Jake's phone started buzzing. It was his mum calling. He declined it.

'Do you want to break up?' Jake said looking genuinely concerned.

'Well, no…' I replied seeing his distraught face, I was unable to remain assertive in my resolve to break up.

'Okay, let's go inside.'

I had to think fast. Jake's phone lit up again. It was his mum.

'No, Jake, go back to your mum's. Take some time and really have a think if this is what you want. I know I'm not fun at the moment, but stick with me, I will get better.'

'Okay. Babe, I love you so much.'

Jake had changed his mind about wanting to break up so quickly that this should've been a red flag. Throughout the relationship, his indecisiveness had always bothered me. Small things like what he wanted to eat, what he wanted to do, and changing plans with friends, always last minute. I went inside and slipped back into bed. Tim was going to be disappointed. I hated disappointing him.

Tim left in the morning, and I didn't tell him about Jake's visit. That day, I was hoping for a big romantic gesture from Jake. Roses. A piece of jewellery. Something. Anything. I secretly wanted things to work out with Jake. I wanted to be loved again. But, two days went by, and I heard nothing. I resisted the urge to call him. I decided it was time to get back into fitness training again. Wearing my snapback cap and my favourite Pokémon T-shirt, I marched down to the gym, determined to get back in shape. I must have looked more like a Pokémon trainer than someone ready to take action. I was feeling good. Towards the end of my workout, Jake walked into the gym. The gym was spacious, but not spacious enough to hide. I could feel my heartbeat quickening. He saw me but did not come over. Okay, what's going on? I went over, and he ignored me coolly until he finished his weight-lifting chest set.

'Er, hi?'

I waved at him to grab his attention.

'Hi.'

To say Jake's response was flat would be an understatement. There was silence in the air, and not the good kind.

I tried again.

'How have you been?'

'Good.'

Wow. Is this all the information I would get out of him?

The conversation felt like it was going nowhere. I said goodbye, turning on my heel to make a quick exit. My sadness and hesitance from that conversation quickly turned into anger. 'Who does he think he is?!' I whipped out my phone and started punching a really angry message to him. Classic old me. These days I'm more able to reflect on the feelings and compose a more thought-out message...well, most of the time.

'You tell me you love me, and you want to get back together, then you ignore me and act as if the other night never happened. What is going on?'

I sent the message. I got a quick reply.

'I don't want to get back together.'

'Fuck.'

I said it out loud, startling a passing stranger. Good thing I lived in London - the Lymington elderly may have had a heart attack. I felt so angry at how he just flip-flopped with this decision. Ever the indecisive Jake. I then broke down crying. Another failed relationship. What is it about me that's causing these relationships to fail? These kinds of thoughts were the first thing that would always pop into my head.

I went back to the flat. I cried. I journaled. I texted my friends. I let out a full-blown scream in anger. I cried some more. I was tempted to dump all his stuff outside by the rubbish bins, but somehow my cooler head prevailed. I calmly composed a text to him.

'I'm going back to my parents for the weekend. Hopefully, it will give you the opportunity to clear your things and leave the key.'

I then blocked his number, deleted him off social media and erased every picture of us together. This felt right. I will give myself time to grieve for this loss, but I will move on. Come out of this better and stronger.

In hindsight, I didn't give myself adequate time to grieve the loss of the relationship. Deleting him from pictures didn't physically delete the relationship. I could feel a knot in my stomach but decided to stick a giant plaster on it. Allowing myself to feel the pain was scary. The emotions were too intense to bear, and thoughts I'd be unlovable forever too overwhelming. But I now understand it's exactly this, the pain of grief, which helps you let go of the old relationship and move on. No matter how strong your grief, it never lasts forever. If I had known how badly I would fall, I would have forced myself to take the time out to grieve.

When I got back from my parents' on Sunday night, all of Jake's things were gone. He left a yellow sticky note with my key saying 'im sorry.' Ugh, this boy. He couldn't even spell 'I'm' correctly. Seriously, what did I see in him? He had even taken the nice bottle of wine we were saving for a special occasion and left his nasty cheap whisky.

Thinking back now, we never really had a serious future. But my mum, my all-knowing guardian, saw this coming from the very beginning. She was right. He was a 'Fun boy', only looking for a good time.

I felt okay at the time, able to brush this breakup off, but it wasn't until my big break down that I truly realised what an impact it had on me and my mental health.

CHAPTER 6

A destructive planet

SATURN

Along with some other stressful events, the post-breakup with Jake eventually led me down a dark road. One of the other events that triggered my depressive state and eventual breakdown was the betrayal of Saturn. Saturn, my then friend and business partner, decided to take everything business-related from me and run away with it - my business plan, my clients and contact lists, my investor. Everything. I had worked for months on the business plan, and she then blocked me from the accounts. I never heard from her again.

Saturn had introduced herself to me at a party in Mayfair. She was wearing a tight-fitting designer dress and expensive high heels. Beautiful dark hair, perfect makeup, red-painted lips, teeth Colgate white and a smile that seemed genuine. She kissed me on the cheek, breath minty, perfume dreamy. She told me she was married, had a rock on her finger to show for it, but that night I saw her leave a party with another man. I found out that she was having multiple affairs. This should have instantly been a red flag, but she explained how her husband mistreated her, and I felt sorry for her.

At the time, I was enamoured by her drive for success and this would blind me to all of the other confusing aspects of her personality. When she suggested we work together, I thought it was a great idea. She was so charming, and I felt myself getting sucked in by the luxury and glamour she surrounded herself with. Picking me up in her sleek black BMW, her polished talons tapping on the wheel to the beat, rolling up to all the VIP parties...I really did like the attention. But by the end of our friendship, I had caught her putting on her multiple identities and picked up her lies, which she would tell compulsively to anyone and everyone around her. Depending on the day of the week, she was either Sharon, Saturn or Samantha. At the end of it all, I couldn't even tell what her name actually was.

She was unreliable as a work colleague and as a friend.

We had just started out gathering clients, and we had snagged a meeting with a potential wealthy client. I had chosen the bar, and Saturn was meant to meet me there an hour before to go through the final notes. The client showed, and Saturn's drink was unaccompanied. To my utter embarrassment, she didn't show up. I smiled and reassured the client she was running late. But she didn't return my calls or messages, and when she did eventually get back to me, there was an excuse. We lost the client. There were always excuses with her. Excuses I believed at first, but soon I began to see patterns. My entire livelihood was hinging on this business, and I needed Saturn to pull her weight. GMK, my godmother, Kate, had warned me about this business relationship, and I reassured her Saturn was a good egg. However, to my frustration, she didn't do any of the work, and I found myself constantly chasing her, only to end up doing the work myself. The business relationship was unbalanced, and when I confronted her about her lies, she went rogue.

Saturn was always golden to my face, but she had said some unpleasant things about me to Jake, which made me feel vulnerable. The friendship was toxic and had a traumatic ending. Confrontation was never a strong point for me, and I was unable to stand my ground when she hurled personal insults at me.

It was she who introduced me to Jake. She said she supported the relationship, but then I discovered after that she had been trying to seduce him.

As my business crumbled, my self-esteem was at an all-time low, and the depression started. Arguments with Jake became more frequent, and instead of turning to new endeavours or exercise, I began comfort eating. I would walk to the shop around the corner, my only movement for that day, and buy dip, crisps and sweets. I spent my days lying on my couch in comfy grey sweats, with my laptop set up for a film or series to lose myself in. I would dispose of the empty wrappers before Jake returned home. Behaving like this every once in a while is okay, but for me, engaging in this kind of behaviour regularly is incredibly unhealthy. My phone buzzed with notifications of messages from friends, but there was nothing in me that wanted to read or reply to them. I didn't want them to know how little I was doing. I found my only communication at that point was with Jake, which must have been tough for him.

My lack of motivation annoyed Jake, and as the pounds started piling on, I started feeling more and more undesirable. A vicious cycle emerged. I was unhappy with my body and comforted myself by eating more, only to feel more unhappy with my body afterwards. I pumped myself with self-loathing, and I became extremely self-conscious, to the point where I couldn't bear to see myself naked, let alone let Jake do so. All of this, on top of my business disintegrating and the betrayal from Saturn, meant my self-worth was at a new low point.

Two of the things I valued in life, having a partner and owning my own business, collapsed. I was in denial about these things coming to an end. There were warnings from my body and my mind, but I chose to ignore them. The knot in my stomach was ever-growing.

Acknowledging the grief and pain inflicted by these endings was a necessary process for a healthy recovery. But I skipped the pain and discomfort. *I'm okay,* I kept saying to myself, ignoring the seeds which had been sowed for my eventual breakdown.

CHAPTER 7

*"Holding on is believing that there's only a past;
letting go is knowing that there's a future" –
Daphne Rose Kingma*

Once I had settled back into the flat, without Jake and without his things, I blitzed the flat clean. I scrubbed the floors and surfaces spotless. Believing I was removing Jake from my soul, satisfaction filled me. I decided to ignore the knot in the pit of my stomach.

'Are you ready to process this hurt?' The knot spoke to me.

'Not today. Today I will sparkle like my kitchen,' I said defiantly.

I jumped on my laptop and started scrolling for PR jobs. Bingo. Central London, Japanese speaker needed, experience preferred. I sent off my CV. My CV was strong, and I nailed interviews. It's always been one of my strengths.

I kept myself busy organising clothes, wardrobes, and throwing away junk collected over the years. It was getting late, and I could no longer put off sleep. I slipped into bed, glancing at the empty space where Jake would have been. I felt a painful pang in my heart.

'Cry,' the pang said to me.

'No. I refuse.' I curled up into a ball, taking up as little space as possible, and after what seemed like hours, finally drifted off to sleep.

When the next morning came, I checked my inbox to see if I had received an interview request. The email that I was hoping for was indeed waiting for me. I congratulated myself. YES. This girl can! I got ready for the gym, and started my day with a bouncy spring in my step.

The interview went well, and I was offered the job on the spot. I was to start working for them the following week. I called Tim, delighted.

'Dinner?' I asked.

'Yes! Japanese food?'

'Always,' I replied.

CHAPTER 8

Am I a cougar???

RYAN

Ryan was incredibly kind, a couple of years younger, and a very handsome master's student in my spin class. I taught at the student gym twice a week before work, and this was where we met. Broad back and strong shoulders, a rugby build with thoughtful eyes, he was articulate and witty. He and his two friends always sat at the front of the class, and I always tried to avoid eye contact with him, as one look from Ryan might lead me to fall off my spin bike. Even though I was in a committed relationship with Jake, I felt a strong force of attraction to Ryan. We had been friends for half a year now, and we shared the same sense of humour. We had hung out a few times outside of class, but I always needed to leave to get home to Jake.

I was getting fitter and eating less as I was socially busy. Food was no longer on my mind as much, long gone the moments I spent binge-eating on my sofa. Dripping in sweat after another fun, pumping spin class, Ryan approached me.

'Hey, do you want to come over for games and drinks?'

'I LOVE games,' I said, smiling.

'Haha, I know you do, see you at 8?'

'Yes, count me in!' I felt excited and had completely forgotten my dinner plans with Tim.

Games night was a hoot. Ryan distracted me from my breakup pain with Jake. He was kind, caring, and as he touched my hand, I looked into his eyes and felt his genuineness. He made me feel special. All thoughts and feelings surrounding Jake melted. It felt like my heart was mending, and upon reflection, although it was only surface level, I was having fun and most importantly, laughing again.

Ryan and I became intimate that evening. For the next couple of weeks, we continued to see each other and we had fun. The truth is, Ryan became part of the giant band-aid for the hurt and rejection from Jake. He was my distraction, and for a while, I felt like things were going to be okay.

It was later, in my darkest moments, to my surprise, Ryan showed up for me in ways Jake never could.

I felt better, having a routine full of exercise and work. I taught spin class, I went to my PR job in central London; on days I wasn't teaching, I met Ryan after work and then would cycle home. I started going out drinking every other evening. This was abnormal behaviour for a person like me who doesn't drink very often. A feeling of recklessness began creeping in. Eating and sleeping were no longer a priority, and there were days I would be functioning on an unhealthy three hours of sleep. Despite my lack of sleep and poor eating habits, I had masses of energy. Looking back, there were warning signs that I was going manic and on the verge of a breakdown. My speech was rapid, I was acting more and more carefree, and I started spending a lot of money. I was on top of the world, untouchable. When my mum called me, I couldn't get my words out fast enough. I became agitated quickly and had masses of sexual energy. I was beyond confident.

Tim and I did end up going out for dinner after I blew him off for Ryan. He had picked an expensive restaurant in central

London. He was dressed in his Armani suit and greeted me with a warm embrace. He then held me at shoulder length, his green eyes looking deep into mine.

'Are you okay? You seem a bit…' Tim trailed off.

'I'm fine, Tim. Actually, I feel great.'

We were shown to our table, and Tim pulled the chair out for me to sit. The lighting was dim, the music romantic and the food delicious. I had a sudden urge to sabotage the atmosphere.

'I'm thinking about experimenting with girls,' I blurted out.

Who knows where this had come from. I later realised the spontaneity was all part of the high I was then experiencing.

'I'm also seeing a master's student, Ryan, he's so much fun and thinks me seeing girls is a great idea.' I was speaking so fast, I was tripping up on my words.

'Okay…as long as you're looking after yourself…are you sure you are okay?' Tim asked worriedly.

'I am more than okay,' I assured, presenting Tim with my winning smile.

THIS GIRL CAN (SOMETIMES)

CHAPTER 9

Work, work, work

The job was peachy at first, and I felt powerful. Strong woman right here. The work building situated in the heart of London Central was swanky. A tall building with glass panels and a swish revolving door. I enjoyed wearing the power suits, red lipstick and charity-find Kurt Geiger black heels. The sound of my heels tapping the floor echoed, and as I swiped my key card to go through, I was always greeted with Colgate smiles from the groomed receptionists. Ryan would visit me on my lunch breaks, I would run to him, and he'd catch me in his arms. Burying the breakup from Jake, I was having a fun time, and I had never felt better. But things turned sour rapidly.

My manager, a robust woman with bobbed frizzy orange hair, always wearing a loud-coloured suit which seemed a bit too snug, gave me a new kind of anxiety. She always wore the same pearl studded earrings to frame her round face and the same bright orange lipstick. She had this Cheshire Cat smile which still haunts me in my dreams today.

I attribute most of my traumatic experiences to her. She made my life difficult, to say the least. It started off with small things. She would pick out flaws in my work and would discipline me for any and all of my mistakes. Charging down the corridor, like a bull that had seen red, colour would rise to her cheeks, and chest puffing out, she would bellow and shout,

35

making an example of me in front of my colleagues. This was her form of 'negative feedback'.

Nothing I did was good enough. If there was a mistake, she would point it out not just to me, but also showcase it in front of my co-workers at the office, so that 'nobody else would make the same basic mistakes'. I had been patiently building my confidence after the breakup with Jake. In a few rounds of workplace humiliation, she was able to tear it all down.

Needless to say, my health began to suffer for it. I started to develop a chesty cough. In most other workplaces, I would have been sent home. But not in this one, and not with this manager. I was told by my manager with an unflinching face, in no uncertain terms, that my health was not a priority here. As I was about to respond, she started shouting at me to pull myself together. I later found out the office next door could hear her shouts. I cried in the toilets but determined not to let it defeat me, I adjusted my makeup and plastered a smile on my face.

I felt constantly manipulated by her.

'My laptop keypad isn't working...' I said one morning.

'Go and replace it then. The Apple store is just around the corner.'

'Okay, I will go after lunch.'

After lunch I got up, ready to leave.

'Where do you think you are going?'

'...to get the keypad fixed?'

'No, work needs to be done.'

'But you said...?'

'No, I didn't.'

I looked at the girls for support, but all heads were down in silence. For all the people that surrounded me every day in this office, I could not have been more alone.

Episodes like these weren't isolated incidents. She made a habit of saying one thing and then an instant later changing her mind. I began doubting myself at every turn. Am I supposed to do this task because she told me to? Or is she going to tell me she never gave me the task and insist I misheard her?

Her constantly-changing positive and negative interactions with me confused me and built on the anxiety. How could someone go from being nice to nasty so quickly? I felt attacked, and my fight or flight system felt permanently switched on if ever she were in the room.

I stopped defending myself. Her routine shouting sessions ended with me hanging my head and apologising for not being good enough. She made me feel like I wasn't good enough.

She had broken me.

One time in particular, I remember crying as I walked home from work after she had shouted in my face that she didn't care whether I lived or died. I felt the whole world crashing around me. Stumbling into people and taking the tube, too unfit to cycle home, I felt all my positive energy had been drained. Could things get any worse? Unfortunately, they did.

To be told by someone that they didn't care whether you lived or died…this must've been the beginning of me losing my mind, literally.

This moment would linger with me for a long time, and it would eventually lead to my breakdown. On the tube home, I received many concerned looks as I sobbed uncontrollably.

My worth had hit rock bottom. I called Han, an old friend, in tears. 'I can't do this anymore,' I sobbed. The line cut out as I went underground.

The box of pain had opened up - Jake, Saturn, the business failing, and my manager's cruelty flooded out in chesty sobs. Through my tears, I saw a man reading The Metro with Andy Murray staring right back at me.

'You're going to be okay.'

'Thanks, Andy,' I said, giving a wobbly smile. The man peered over the newspaper, caught my eye, and quickly looked away.

I was pretty sure my boss had asked one of the girls to take my work notebook, which documented all the horrible things she had said to me, from my bag as I never found it again. It is important for people to feel trust, worth and connection in order to grow and thrive. In this workplace, though, I could find no traces of that anywhere I looked. This is when my paranoia really set in, and I couldn't be sure what was real. I couldn't tell who my friends were. It started to feel like everyone was out to get me.

Ryan tried his best to support me, noticing my volatile moods. I went out of my way to be extra outgoing during dinner and insisted we go clubbing on weeknights. He tried to ask about work, but I wouldn't engage - I didn't want to let him in to help me. I feared he wouldn't want to see me anymore if I wasn't 'fun'. I didn't want him to abandon me like Jake had. He, as well as my friends, noticed my spike in energy and me dropping large amounts of money for dinner and drinks. They also picked up on my more outgoing, sometimes outrageous behaviour, but no one could have predicted it was the beginning of my mania.

I had to get out of that job. With help from Alistair, a close friend, who supported me through countless encouraging phone calls, I wrote the resignation email. I managed to leave.

CHAPTER 10

"The friend who can be silent with us in a moment of despair or confusion, who can stay with us in an hour of grief and bereavement, who can tolerate not knowing…not healing, not curing…that is a friend who cares" – Henri Nouwen

ALISTAIR - A-SAN

Dear A-San

Remember when I gave you this nickname at our first working event? I was working for a Japanese company and added 'san' at the end of your name, a Japanese sign of respect, and I gave myself the nickname Tiger Fang over the walkie talkies.

You have become one of my dearest and closest friends. Always a logical and practical person, you have an appropriate answer for everything.

With your glasses, an all-knowing genuine smile and analytical mind, you have been through thick and thin with me. After another breakup (before Jake), I was distraught, and you sent me twelve gifts, one to open every day to help me get through the breakup. Your gifts included things that sparked joy or interest. On day three, I opened a box of modelling clay. I created aliens and magical creatures, making a slow-motion

*picture. Your last note and gift said, 'You can get through this',
and you were right.*

*After my breakup from Jake and hard time at work, I came
home to find a beautiful vase of flowers you had delivered,
which once again ignited a light within me.*

*I am so grateful we have stayed in touch since 2013. It was
thanks to you that I was able to publish my first book, 'Hare
and Tortoise Have Counselling', and my children's book, 'The
Hafu Child'.*

*Without you, I wouldn't have been able to get through the
really rough times. In my breakdown, you tried talking to me
on the phone, you visited me in the institute and brought me
puzzles to help me with my anxiety.*

*You are one of my biggest supporters in all my interests
and work. You are always there to help me with any practical,
technical or life issues; you helped me build my fitness and
work website. I can't thank you enough.*

Love, your friend for life.

Tiger Fang

CHAPTER 11

The building of a crescendo

I left the PR job when I was 26.

Mum was worried about me. She'd seen my mental health deteriorate before. There was a time she flew out to Japan, where I was studying during my year abroad, to help me through an eating disorder. She tends to know when I'm not doing well. My phone calls to her in this time had felt similar to those times in Japan. However, I was doing a desperate job of convincing her I was fine.

I became overly agitated and unable to sleep through the night. I would wake up, sweat dripping down my back, and my breathing rapid. But when morning came, I was buzzed to start the day, an unnatural energy after all those sleepless nights. The nights became my nemesis, always leaving me in anguish. Mum insisted I come home, trying to suggest it carefully so I wouldn't hear the worry in her voice.

She hoped a trip to Lymington would allow my body and mind to relax and recharge. It was what I desperately needed.

I caught the train back to Lymington. Standing in Waterloo station, I felt elevated, beyond happy. Waterloo always reminded me of train trips to and from home, and I loved the open space and airy feel of the station. Having just had dinner with Ryan, I felt he was a definite keeper. A couple of nights of good sleep at home in Lymington and everything will be fine. 'I'm fine,' I kept telling myself. Not realising I was muttering this out loud, the person next to me looked uncomfortable. I smiled at him and looked away, convincing myself I just needed to rest. Ryan and I had made fun plans for the next week, and I couldn't wait. I looked up and saw a pigeon perched on the clock, flapping its wings. Feeling like this pigeon had acknowledged me, I nodded back smiling. The person beside me looked more uncomfortable. They announced the platform to my train, and I made my way there. 'See you in two days, Ms Waterloo Station!'

Little did I know it would be months until my next return to London.

The train ride had been smooth - exchanging messages with Ryan, big headphones on, bopping my head to my music. Looking back, I didn't realise my constant need for engagement. I couldn't sit still, fingers tapping away non-stop on my phone, eyes glued to the screen. Music so loud it blocked out all thinking. This didn't feel healthy.

I arrived at Brockenhurst Station and was greeted by mum and my dog, Luffy. I took a quick selfie with Luffy in the car, and sent it to Ryan, uploaded it to my Instagram, captioning it - good to be home with my favourite dog. It ended up being my last post for a long time.

A deceiving paranoia began setting in. Arriving home, I tucked myself up on the sofa, green tea at my side, and opened up the local newspaper. I started seeing hidden messages. I moved to the wooden floor, crouched down and spread the paper in front of me. Smoothing it over with my hands, I saw an article headlined 'Cancer is back'. I reread and reread those three words. Wait. Is this newspaper telling me mum is unwell? I sensed my uneasiness and confusion. I hugged my knees in, making myself small. I rocked my whole body slightly. I then looked up and stared at mum, who was now sitting on the sofa.

'Mum, everything okay?'

THIS GIRL CAN (SOMETIMES)

'Yes.' She smiled.

'Are you okay?'

'I'm fine,' she said, looking up from her paper.

I asked again, 'Are you sure?'

'Yes…' mum had stopped reading, seeming concerned.

'Promise me you aren't lying to me?' mum met my intense look.

'Yes, I'm fine…are you okay?'

I broke eye contact, 'Yes, all well with me,' I said in a chipper voice. I abruptly got up, and crumpling the newspaper, I threw it in the recycling. 'My mind must be playing tricks on me,' I muttered, shaking my head slightly.

I stepped outside and took some deep breaths. The sky had turned a murky grey which matched the mood of my clouded mind. I unlocked my Corsa, sat in the driver's seat and turned on the radio. Eyes closed, I drummed my finger on the steering wheel to the beat. As the song ended, the radio presenter announced casually, 'God is always watching you.' I opened my eyes, frowning. How odd. Since when did Radio 1 start making bold statements like that? The presenter then called out my first name. I switched it off instantly. Feeling confused, my mind seemed to be deteriorating throughout the day. It's as if my brain had caged me and I couldn't get past my overly suspicious thoughts.

Stepping out of the car, I called Luffy and decided a walk around the Sea Wall would help clear my mind. The Sea Wall is an 18km stone path, and a lovely walk around the marshes, which can take you to Keyhaven Sailing Club or the Lymington Sailing Club. Walking past the Salterns, a saltwater lake separated from the sea by the Sea Wall, I halted and stared at the sailing club. I had learnt to sail here as a child, and I tried to let those fond memories wash over me. My dog Luffy sat patiently by my side. I heard my name being called. Just my imagination, I thought, but when I opened my eyes, I saw some

43

family friends. I greeted them energetically but was having difficulty following the conversation. I soon trailed off, unable to finish my sentence. Words had abandoned me. I looked towards the sky. Clouds were flying by with immense speed. A little confused, they politely said goodbye, mentioning how nice it was to see me. The encounter had felt surreal, as if I had made it up.

Later on in the year, if those family friends hadn't brought up how different I was behaving in that encounter, I would have believed I had made it up.

Still planted on the same spot, what felt like seconds were actually minutes. Luffy started to whine, bringing me back to this reality. I reached for my phone and saw the message pop up in red: 'DANGER'. Unable to finish the walk, we turned back. Luffy, trying to keep up with my brisk pace, looked up at me. We made eye contact, and even he looked worried.

I was alert and on edge for the rest of the day. I could barely eat. I didn't look at my phone after the danger message. I found myself pacing around the house, eyes cast down, occasionally rubbing the sides of my arms.

JIGSAW MELTDOWN

That night, I was sitting on the floor in the living room, calmly doing a jigsaw puzzle with the television on in the background. I started hearing voices. Low volume at first, but as I concentrated, I recognised the voices. My old friends and ex-boyfriend from university were talking to me through the television. My back was turned to the screen so I couldn't see them, but I was certain they were all behind me.

'HEY! Come outside, we are all waiting for you!'

I started to laugh, and they began cheering me on to leave the house. Hastily standing up, I rushed upstairs and packed a small bag, ready to leave. My university boyfriend, James, was outside, ready to take me away. My friends missed me, they still cared about me and everything was going to be okay. James wanted to get married and was deeply sorry for breaking my heart. Dad, confused by my actions, had to quickly block the doorway to stop me from leaving the house.

'Dad, get out of my way, he's waiting for me outside!'

'But who is waiting for you outside?'

'James, of course! He proposed to me through the television.'

'Let's go back inside and talk.' My dad quickly realised he had to enter my fantasy world to get me to stay inside.

'It's late, shall we go to sleep and see how you feel tomorrow?'

'But James…'

'…James will wait.' It was at this moment dad became overwhelmed with panic and sadness that I was no longer myself.

It's interesting my mind took me back to James and my university friends. I hadn't thought about them over the years, and the breakup with James had been traumatic after he confessed to seeing someone else during my year abroad in Japan.

I went to bed, but sleep didn't visit me. I lay in bed, eyes wide open, feeling confused about what had happened earlier that evening. Reality and fantasy were head to head in battle. The line of truth was blurring. Not sleeping turned out to be one of the key factors for my mental health falling apart so rapidly. Tossing and turning, my phone lit up as I received messages, some from real people, some not. A crackling noise played on loop in my mind. The TV, although switched off, began talking to me. 'Don't trust your family,' and spurred on my feelings of anxiety and paranoia.

Darkness pulled away any remaining light within me. Evoked by a new kind of menacing fear, I was left terrified and believing these paranoias. I felt isolated. The feeling of 'trust no one' pulsed through me. Inanimate objects talking to me became my new normal, and I accepted their whisperings.

2am, after a restless short sleep, I awoke and I tried to do the jigsaw puzzle again. If I complete the jigsaw puzzle, the truth will be revealed. My hands shaking, body jittering, I couldn't fit any of the pieces together. My hands weren't obeying me. Someone had increased the colour contrast of the jigsaw pieces. I rubbed my eyes, brain hurting. I threw the puzzle box across the room and started pacing once again, muttering to myself. 'I need a pen. I need to map this out.'

So I started drawing on the wall. I began mind-mapping my paranoia, convinced it stemmed from the breakup with Jake, business partner Saturn, and my horrible boss. Arrows flew out everywhere. Everyone was out to get me. I started hearing sirens outside. When morning came, and my parents and brother saw my bedroom wall covered in scribbles and paranoid theories, stunned and worried, they couldn't speak.

I backed away from them, calling Ryan. 'I'm not crazy!' Putting him on speakerphone. 'Ryan believes me! Ryan, tell them I'm not crazy.' I started to sob. My brother calmly said, 'Okay, we believe you,' taking the phone off me.

GMK

I went to stay with GMK (Godmother Kate). My mum thought the stability of the farm and the close relationship I had with GMK might help bring me back into reality. I stepped

THIS GIRL CAN (SOMETIMES)

out onto their patio and absorbed the view of green fields and the wandering farm animals. The farm feels free and is a true reflection of GMK. Her spirit is free.

My godmother is superwoman. A doctor, smart, fun and loving, she is someone I have always looked up to, and I felt safe in her presence. But being at the farm, there wasn't much improvement. Sat in the living room, GMK tried playing some music, but I found the modern beats too stressful. She quickly switched to classical music, noticing my body tense. I hugged my knees in, mind disorientated. I was able to converse at a normal level, but then I would start tailing off, unable to finish my sentences once again. I couldn't engage in any activity. GMK and her daughter Vita tried to get me involved in some yoga and exercises, but I remained on the sofa, silent. I was also silent at the dinner table. I couldn't concentrate on anything, words felt like they were slipping away from me, and I couldn't catch them. It felt like a slippery frog was jumping around in my mind, and I couldn't quite catch it.

GMK thought it would be a good idea to keep my phone for me. But without it, I felt even more vulnerable. Before putting me to bed, she read me and her other two children a bedtime story.

I'm safe, I thought, and closed my eyes, but as if my brain was being scraped by a cheese grater, my eyes snapped wide open. I felt wired, and the fear sank in as I realised sleep would once again not be visiting me.

The next morning, I came downstairs full of energy and asked George, GMK's husband, if I should wake the kids up to go for a run. He looked at me sadly, 'It's a school morning.'

'Oh, right, silly me.' I sat down at the wooden table and pretended to read. But the letters were jumbled up. I squeezed my eyes shut and opened them again, the magazine now stated 'RUN, and you will be fine'.

'I'm going for a run.'

THIS GIRL CAN (SOMETIMES)

'Why not try a walk? Go around the fields,' George smiled encouragingly. I stepped out onto the grounds, swinging my arms slightly. I'm fine. But catching sight of a concrete wall connecting the barn filled me with agitation and an unwelcome dread. My chest tightened, and I felt trapped. I tried to make my way to the fields, but it was as if I was stuck in a maze, with only me in it. The sun was warm on my face, but I quickly became too warm, and I could feel sweat start to slide down my back. I headed back to the house.

CHAPTER 12

Losing my marbles

My godmother took me home, and mum answered the door. They exchanged words. Their lips were moving, but I could only hear the white, fuzzy noise on loop. GMK left, and I walked into the kitchen. Stood in the middle, the blue-painted countertops glowed, feeling more vibrant than I remembered. Everything felt a little too bright. Then it came to me, a moment of clear clarity.

I turned to mum with an intent stare, stating, 'Mum, we need to stay in the house.'

I had become convinced we couldn't leave the house as we may be spotted.

'Spotted by who?' mum said worriedly.

'I'm not sure, but I know we can't leave right now.'

'Okay, why don't you take a rest?'

I moved to the sofa, but couldn't rest. I was talking to myself and found myself once again pacing.

GMK came back later to take me to my GP. It was a struggle to get me to leave the house as my mind was breaking down rapidly. The beginning of my full mental breakdown. I literally lost my mind. I believed I was Angelina Jolie, and the paparazzi were after me. I wore sunglasses in the car and kept my head low. Arriving at the practice, I began to stick my leg out just like Angelina Jolie had done in that famous photo.

'What are you doing?' GMK asked.

'I'm working it. The paparazzi love me,' I said, flashing my teeth and angling my legs. I removed my godmother's silk scarf and wrapped it around me. 'I need to show off my best side!' It must have looked completely bizarre in practice, sticking my leg out to random people. I was greeted with some very bewildered looks.

GMK took me back home to my parents after I remembered vaguely seeing my GP. She had touched my forehead, flashed a light in my eyes and asked me how I was, to which I responded, 'Just peachy!' GMK calmly explained the situation and that I needed to be seen by the mental health team. My GP could not do much at this point, aside from arranging for someone from the psychiatric department to visit the house to assess me. But nobody came. Things were difficult as I was over 18, and there seemed to be a serious lack of funding in the system.

My mum, unable to cope, called Jonathon, GMK's father, and a retired doctor. He had been a family friend for a long time and came over instantly. Mum was desperate.

I have a clear memory of Jonathon coming to the house. Things had been pretty blurry up until that point. What I thought was a 5-minute visit was actually a 5-hour one. I believed Jonathon was Jake, just older. He had the same piercing blue eyes.

'DON'T COME NEAR ME!' I kept crying and shouting at him. 'YOU HURT ME.' Things were getting worse. I started to become more violent, flinging my arms around, trying to sit up and push past Jonathon. In my mind I wasn't crazy, they were crazy. Everything felt so real, I couldn't understand why everyone around me seemed so panicked. I was in danger.

We were told that we would get a visit from the mental health unit to assess the situation. But as the day passed no word came from anybody - my parents had no choice but to take me to A&E, the emergency services. I remember the journey vividly.

'Mum, we are being chased!' I said, trying to peer out the window.

'No, we are okay, we are safe,' mum said, concerned as she tried to get me to sit back.

I was so sure at the time that we were being chased by someone. For what, I didn't care to even think about. My mum brought Luffy. She placed him right next to me in an attempt to keep me calm.

'Stroke Luffy, he will keep you safe,' mum said, trying to smile. Little did I know the weight of her worry behind that smile.

Sitting in the waiting room, I began rubbing my hand on my left leg whilst bouncing my right fist on the other leg, then switching over to the other leg. In my mind, it was a survival mechanism - I needed to do this to stay alive. I remember a man sat opposite me crossing his legs, and I began mirroring his actions. He realised what I was doing and moved to another seat. The lights in the waiting room started flashing, telling me, 'Saturn, Jake, your boss, they are all out to get you!' It was a surreal experience.

What happened after is a fuzzy memory. Two doctors and one social worker were required to assess me in order to section me. However, A&E could not get hold of anyone until the next day.

I was sedated to help me remain calm, and stayed the night in the hospital.

They had put me in a children's ward room. Appropriate, as I had regressed into a childlike state. I remember animals all over the wall. I began pairing the animals up, and Mum started helping me. Dad spotted an animal which didn't have a partner and pointed this out which immediately caused me distress.

'John! We had just calmed her down!' mum exclaimed to my dad.

'Sorry,' dad hung his head. Mum tried to soothe me and put me to sleep. They stayed by my side and comforted me. All would be well. Poor Luffy had to sleep in the car by himself.

I don't remember how I got there or who took me, but mum told me an ambulance transferred me from A&E to the mental health institute. My next clear memory was waking up in a cramped room. It was a tough time for my parents, as being over 18, I had to admit myself, but apparently, I refused to read the letter or sign the paperwork to admit myself. I kept throwing it back at them, which seems very comical now. Mum had to hold her hand over mine to help sign my name.

In the institution, there were rows of small bedrooms, very much like dorms or halls at a university accommodation. There was a musty smell, and it was all very brown. Whoever designed the colour scheme must have loved the colour brown, as it was everywhere. Doors, furniture, carpets, even some of the paintings. People walked around dressed in comfortable clothing, but I saw them all as dangerous strangers. I understand these places are a necessity for people mentally unfit to live and be by themselves, but this was no hotel and not a nice place to be. Anyone who remotely looked like Jake or Saturn sent me into a panic. I kept to myself.

My parents were able to visit me and go into my small room to make sure I was okay. I was grateful for this, as I felt very scared and lonely, often in tears for fear of sleeping. It's always just before I go to bed, just before I sleep, that immense fear creeps in. Fear of being left with my thoughts. And during that time, and still even at times now, my thoughts can scare me.

There were many characters in this institute. I remember one particular person, a pregnant woman struggling with

THIS GIRL CAN (SOMETIMES)

bipolar. She scared me. She talked to me with her face inches from mine. I winced as spit flew from her mouth. She said I needed to watch myself, they were always watching. But who was always watching? I became paranoid that people such as Saturn and Jake were watching me. It is clear now, looking back, she had a range of different mental health issues and me being exposed to her and others in the institute, did nothing to improve mine. It had a negative knock-on effect, and I felt I was absorbing the paranoia.

At one point, I believed Sir Alex Ferguson, the former Man United football manager, had come to visit me in the small garden at the institute. I had worked at a sports media company before starting my own company, and always liked how he did his interviews. I was put on a lot of drugs, heavy drugs, enough drugs to stop the hallucinations. The managers of the institute also found me unpredictable and a potential risk to myself, so I was assigned a helper.

'Who are you talking with?' asked the helper.

'Well, Sir Alex Ferguson, of course. I have just interviewed him for an exclusive piece on what his expectations are for the Japanese player, Shinji Kagawa,' I smiled back.

'Well, that is exciting!' the helper retorted.

I don't remember the helper's name, but she had an impact on my stay. She kept me safe and gave me comfort. She entered my world with me as she soon discovered I became very distressed if she couldn't see what I could see.

In my time at the institute, I stole a chess piece. It's like my spinning top. In the 2010 movie, Inception, Leonardo DiCaprio's character experiences hallucinations, and he spins a top to help him figure out whether he is in the real world or not. For me, it was a chess piece. I refused to give it back, believing it was important to establish I was not in a parallel universe. So in the end, they let me keep it. I would hold it at all times, just like the top Leonardo DiCaprio held onto. This is a piece I still have today. Whenever I feel anxious, reaching for it in my pocket helps me relieve the anxiety, and with the logical left side of my brain being activated, I can focus on the sensation of touch. If I ever feel myself becoming anxious, I tune into my senses. I then find it easier to question my thoughts objectively.

The women's lounge was daunting. I felt anxious being around them, not quite keeping up with any of their conversations. I convinced myself it was best to go undercover and pretend to be a boy to stay safe. My life depended on it.

I ended up being asked to leave the institute as I kept wandering over to the boys' wing. Curling up into a ball on their sofa, I felt more comfortable on the boys' side. The pregnant woman scared me, and I felt there was less noise on this side.

'Mum, I'm a boy. It's fine!' I would tell her.

'No, you're a girl,' she would respond calmly.

'I think I would know!' Nonsensical conversations like this would be part and parcel of my manic episode.

Both Ryan and Alistair came to visit me. I knew who they were, but I was still in the depths of a manic episode. I remember that I kept doing the Hunger Games tribute, hand up in the air, whistling the Mockingjay tune. I pretended to faint once to avoid being taken back to the women's dorms. Ryan had to pick me up and take me to my room where I tried to convince him he could stay with me as we were both boys.

Alistair had brought a new jigsaw puzzle, but I was restless, constantly walking in and out of the room. I tried to fit jigsaw pieces together, sometimes successfully, other times not. My hands trembled with agitation, and I went to open the window as heat rose to my face. I longed to open the window wide, consume some fresh air, but the lock meant it could only open a little way. The room felt too warm. Sweat sliding down the back of my arms, I took my jumper off, only to put it on again. I was acting frantic and being indecisive, but Alistair didn't panic or compulsively check in to see if I was okay. He sat on the chair and continued to do the jigsaw puzzle, occasionally peering over his glasses to find the next piece. The act was grounding. I eventually calmed enough to sit beside him and continue the jigsaw puzzle with him. The silence was no longer deafening, feelings of agitation easing as we worked.

When Alistair left, sleep came to me easily for the first time.

During one of our routine check-ins, the head of the institute decided it was best if I was transferred to another institute. He thought it might be less triggering for me. By the time I was transferred, the drugs were really kicking in, and I was slowly coming back to reality. I felt groggy, but I knew who I was again, I was aware of the situation, and I now wanted to go home. They did not permit family in my room at the new institution, so I felt very scared and alone.

The room itself was small and dank, with the bed feeling hard. The walk to the shower room was daunting, as anyone could see you. Mum had bought me some new clothes, so I would change into my grey tracksuit bottoms and grey jumper after taking a lukewarm shower, and shuffle back quickly to my small, dark room.

This place was just as hard as the last place. In my mind, a recovery centre is white space, yoga, white linen clothes, spas…this was not my experience being in these mental health institutes. They were dark, dingy, and I did not feel comfortable or at home. The space was crowded, small, and I felt scared being alone and not knowing anyone.

Mum and dad visited me every day, signing me out to go on walks and have meals at restaurants. I don't remember this, but my mum told me later that my dad broke down quite a bit

THIS GIRL CAN (SOMETIMES)

before and after these visits. I have rarely seen my dad cry. My mum really had to keep it together.

'Will she ever be herself again?' dad asked mum in the car, having just visited me.

'Yes, but you need to be strong. Pull yourself together,' mum said with strong resolve.

I was allowed my mobile back and only talked to two people. Mum and Tim. Tim would call to check in. He had been in frequent contact with mum about how I was doing. He became my lifeline to the outside world, and my feelings for him started changing from friendship to something more. On the phone, I acted as if I was fine, and my breakdown had actually never happened. Tim always kept the conversation positive and encouraged me to start some exercise again. Mum suggested I started drawing again, something I had always enjoyed growing up.

So, I began exercising and painting. I talked to other patients in the ward, including a patient I called Penguin, like the character from Batman. He dressed like him, carried an umbrella which he would swing about, laughing all the way. That part, I know, was real.

I looked forward to being able to leave. Escape the other patients. I don't know where I would be without my family and Alistair coming to see me. Their visits kept me connected to the outside world, believing that one day I would be released from this institute where I felt trapped, and be able to re-join my friends and family.

When mum and dad took me out to pubs and restaurants, they were encouraging me to eat; my clothes fitting a little too loosely. How fragile I had become. Face pale, hands clasped on my lap, I would be shivering despite it being a warm day. Eyes cast down, I couldn't make conversation, and my confidence had plummeted. Worries embedded in my parents' faces, they would smile encouragingly and discuss Luffy, the weather, and anything else that came to mind to avoid the silence.

Alistair came and signed me out to take me to the cinema. Fortunately, it was only us in the screening. Sat back in the plush chair, it started off with me drumming my fingers on my lap, then came the shaking of my foot. Overwhelmed with too much darkness and my mind feeling like it could explode, I surrendered to my need to jump up and move around. I had managed 15 minutes seated watching the film. I got up and paced around the cinema for the remaining 60 minutes. It was like watching some caged animal. Alistair remained in his seat, allowing me to pace with no judgement.

After the cinema, we sat in a restaurant. The background noises fuelled my anxiety. I was still hearing the crackly white noise on loop in my mind. Alistair noticed my face scrunching up and touched my hand, his face showing genuine concern. At that moment, the background noise diminished, and it was like someone was tuning the radio in my mind. Then came this stunning clarity. I closed my eyes. I could hear my breathing, feel my chest rise and fall. I opened my eyes, and I could finally see. I knew who I was.

I felt dread as Alistair drove me back to the institute. It was dinner time, and at mealtimes, I always sat alone at the tables. Nobody really wanted to interact with me. The food was very bland. It wasn't enough I had to deal with the mania and hallucinations of football managers; I also had to deal with mushy vegetables. One eventful mealtime, a girl grabbed her table knife and threatened to kill the person next to her, and I knew I had to jump through all the hoops and do anything it took to get out of this place. I could manage feelings of loneliness, but fear fed into my anxiety, hindering my recovery.

I still didn't look healthy, and I was not permitted to go home until they deemed me mentally fit. I was still losing weight and was suffering from tremors. The psychologist was hard to get meetings with, and in my first meeting upon entering the institute, I told him my conspiracy theories. I was nervous about us meeting again, worried he might not see me fit to leave, but after the table knife incident, I insisted on meeting with him again. This was the meeting where I needed to convince him I was ready to leave. I looked at the window in the room, thinking maybe I could plan my escape here and now. I clearly remember him in his chair looking very pensive. He was an elderly man who looked tired, so, really, he could have just fallen asleep. I made my case, and he eventually made the decision I was able to leave.

CHAPTER 13

Into recovery we go

I was almost 27 when I was allowed home. At long last. But being on such heavy medication, I couldn't even tie my own shoes, let alone go out and cross the road. I couldn't read. My eyes blurred every time I tried to focus on the words.

Mum and I practised relaxation in the mornings, where I would inhale and isolate, engage different muscle groups then exhale, relaxing. This was an incredibly calming exercise, but occasionally my body would start shaking uncontrollably, spreading through me until it looked like I was having a seizure. Tears streaming down my face, mum had to quickly place her hands on my shoulders, telling me to breathe until the shaking stopped.

My body was not connecting with my brain, meaning my body wasn't telling me when I needed to use the bathroom. I could no longer fall asleep by myself anymore. Mum had to wait in the room until I fell asleep. But despite my new anxiety around travelling, I still insisted on some normality and continued to go up to London to return and teach my two spin classes. Teaching exercise I found relieving - with the music loud and body engaged, my mind had no time to wonder. I would also see Ryan there and tried to see Tim as often as possible.

I had trouble with sitting, reading, and watching films. The concentration made me feel overly anxious. Travelling on the train, I was very agitated. Mum accompanied me on all my trips to London. On the train journeys, she had to give me bits of rubbish to keep putting in the bin so I could get up and move.

When I saw Ryan, he could see I was unwell, and with his final master's exams coming up, he had to take a step back. He was not in the position to commit to a relationship, and although sad at the time, I understood that he needed to do what was best for him.

My sadness quickly turned into anger, a slow rage filling my throat until I couldn't breathe. I was angry for being unwell. I was angry that I could no longer do anything without my mum being at my side. I had regressed to a child. This illness had me losing Ryan and left me fragile and weak.

CHAPTER 14

Bipolar, the facts

So, I was diagnosed with bipolar. According to bipolaruk.org, around one to two percent of people will develop bipolar disorder, formerly known as manic depression. People with bipolar disorder will experience both episodes of severe depression, and episodes of mania — overwhelming joy, excitement, happiness, huge energy, a reduced need for sleep, and reduced inhibitions.

The experience of bipolar is uniquely personal. It was interesting to discover that no two people have exactly the same experience.

Bipolar disorder has been associated with genius and with creativity. Throughout history, it is possible to recognise bipolar personality traits in the artistic, political and academic spheres. For example, Mariah Carey, Stephen Fry, Mel Gibson, and my best friend Selena Gomez has also recently shared her bipolar traits. But what is bipolar actually?

The exact cause of bipolar disorder is still unknown. But experts believe there are a number of factors that work together to make a person more likely to develop it. These are thought to be a complex mix of physical, environmental and social factors.

These types of life-altering events can cause episodes of depression at any time in a person's life. There can be many triggers, but for me, stress and lack of sleep were my key triggers.

There is some evidence that if there is an imbalance in the levels of one or more neurotransmitters, a person may develop some symptoms of bipolar disorder. For example, there is evidence that episodes of mania may occur when levels of noradrenaline are too high, and episodes of depression may be the result of noradrenaline levels becoming too low.

It is also thought that bipolar disorder is linked to genetics, as it often runs in families. The family members of a person with bipolar disorder have an increased risk of developing it themselves. But no single gene is responsible for bipolar disorder. Instead, a number of genetic and environmental factors are thought to act as triggers. No one in my family has had mental health issues like I have.

Thinking of bipolar as highs and lows is too simplistic. This disorder is complex, unique and layered. The best way to explain it is that I have a chemical imbalance in the brain where my neurotransmitters are off their game due to the severe mental break. People feel sadness, yes, but for me, having bipolar means when I feel sad, it quickly dips into a very dark place, and sometimes I feel suicidal. On good days, I choose life, on bad days, I choose the imaginary red pill. A pill which could send me to an eternal sleep.

MEDICATION

I hated being on medication, but it was necessary as my symptoms were severe, and my behaviour would become extremely disturbing without it. From the heavy dose of different coloured pills, my medication was changed to Aripiprazole, a mood stabiliser, and Clonazepam, a pill to help me sleep. For me, and others like me who are deep into recovery and need medication, it's about keeping an eye on the situation, understanding that taking medication doesn't make you weak.

For many, if not most people with bipolar, life and keeping well includes taking medication. This is something I can finally now accept. The thing I prioritise most with keeping myself well is to be strict in taking my medication. I figured out pretty quickly, missing doses or tweaking them without professional help had devastating effects.

Even while being on heavy medication, it took almost an entire year to be able to sit still for longer than 5 minutes. It was tough being that anxious and agitated all the time. Sadness always led to feelings of fury. I needed then, more than ever, to be kind to myself. Forgive my body, forgive my mind, and love and accept myself as I was in that moment.

I am grateful for my psychotherapist, Dr Jean Rias. She monitored the medication, counselled me through the experience, and was the first to tell me of my bipolar diagnosis. I was defensive meeting her for the first time, arms crossed like a stroppy teenager, but she built trust quickly. Counsellors I had encountered up until meeting her had lacked empathy, but Dr Jean Rias had an abundance of this. Her body language was open and always neutral, her voice calm. Her shoulder-length brown hair framed her dark eyes and warm smiles. You couldn't help but like her.

I was in denial about having bipolar for the longest time. It must have been a good two years until I was able to get over the stigma associated with someone with a mental condition like mine. I rejected the idea of it and told no one about the situation.

I threw myself fully into treatment to get well. Through Dr Jean Rias, I learned some good strategies for taking care of myself. If ever you're struggling with mental health, remember there's an individual under the diagnosis. There was a 'you' before you were diagnosed, and there will be one after.

Bipolar might have changed me, but that's okay. I consider myself to be on a journey involving acceptance and recovery. Recovery doesn't necessarily mean I'm okay or I'm cured, but it can mean new opportunities. Without the journey and recovery, I wouldn't be writing this book. That's for sure.

CHAPTER 15

Understanding what had happened

Dr Jean Rias explained that what I experienced in London was a manic episode with psychotic symptoms. I sat back in the chair and absorbed her words.

'Can you tell me about a time you felt sad?' she asked.

Memories of me lying in bed, unable to get up post-breakup came flooding back.

After talking about this memory, and my life up until London, it turned out that I had experienced depressive episodes previously in my life. But never manic.

Upon reflection, I would always be in a vicious cycle of getting boyfriends, getting dumped, falling into depression, and then getting triggered by something that would inspire me to start getting fit again. But I would repeat the process and find a new boyfriend, get dumped, gain weight, get depressed, etc.

However, in London it was different. Triggered by life events: a breakup, a broken business and a toxic workplace, my mania lasted for three weeks. Building up speed and momentum to that breakdown point, the lack of sleep put my brain into overdrive. Above all, unable to relax or rest was crippling for the mind and body. After that manic episode and coming back to reality, I felt unhappy and ashamed about how I had behaved.

Why did I tell Tim that I was experimenting with women? Why did I collapse on the floor pretending to be so delicate when Ryan came to visit me in the hospital?

I kept the mental breakdown and one-month disappearance a secret from my friends. They thought I just went off the radar and had come back slimmer. When seeing my friends, it was always for an activity, either walking or cycling together. I recall going for coffee and finding it incredibly difficult.

'Are you okay?' my friend asked.

'Yes, fine, why?' I said, smiling.

'Your foot seems to be in overdrive.' I looked down to see my foot bouncing up and down. I was feeling anxious. I checked my watch again, I'd only been sitting here for two minutes and already I wanted to get up and leave.

'Do you have ADHD or something?'

'No,' I said, laughing. The coffee shop was getting busier. My palms started to feel clammy, heat rising to my cheeks.

'I'm getting the worst cramps.' I stood up abruptly. 'Do you mind if we walk for a bit?'

'Sure.' She looked concerned.

As we walked outside, I gulped down the cool air. My chest loosened. When will this end? Throat tight, I held back my tears. Being able to sit and have coffee with a friend should never be taken for granted.

Life became militant. I went to bed at 9pm and woke up at 6am every day. I needed a clear routine and structure to my day. I started my day with stretching and breathing exercises, followed by a walk in the park with Luffy whilst talking to Alistair on the phone. I would come home, have breakfast, and write out my day with set times for each activity, so every moment was occupied. I allocated slots for attempted downtime. It was these times I dreaded the most.

CHAPTER 16

Birthday surprise

Tim had gone out of his way to travel two hours from London to see me for my birthday. I felt very special that day. I picked him up from the station, and we embraced like lovers would do. I took him out on the rib, his laugh getting lost in the wind as we sped over the waves. We had a roast at the sailing club with my family after. I felt like myself pre-bipolar diagnosis. Carefree, not controlled by my tight time schedule, and able to laugh and have fun again.

The next day, on my birthday, he presented me with a silver ring that I had spotted at Greenwich Market months ago. I commented on it, tried it on and put it back, feeling it was too expensive. He must have gone back to buy it after we parted.

He had stood by me throughout an incredibly dark time in my life, and he never gave up trying to contact me and support me. My feelings for him had only strengthened throughout my time in hospital and in recovery. At this point, I was in love with Tim. I had written him a letter saying that he had always been something more than a friend, and my love for him was deeper than the surface level love I had for Jake. It took time for me to have the courage to read him my letter. I stood in front of him, hands trembling as I held the piece of paper, my voice wavering at times as he listened intently. After I'd finished reading, he thanked me for my letter. I waited. That was it.

'It's getting late, let's go to sleep,' he said. So, we got ready for bed.

I watched him sleep, his back turned to me. Wasn't this what he had wanted? Didn't he love me back? I lay awake, replaying his reaction. Had I expected too much?

After a walk around the park together the next morning, I dropped him back at the station. The letter wasn't mentioned once. We embraced goodbye, but something felt off. I reassured myself that he was just concerned about his new business and eager to get back to continue working.

Tim went back to London, and I started work again. I tried to continue with my life like the rejection from my letter never happened.

CHAPTER 17

I'll be up in the gym, just working on my fitness

FITNESS AND MY CLIENTS – HUSTLE HARD

My PUMP IT UP playlist is on full blast. My Bluetooth headphones are blocking the outside world. It's just me running around the Sea Wall. I visualise myself in a film where the lead needs to train for a big event. I'm singing out loud to the words. My body feels strong, my breathing in rhythm with my running steps. I'm by no means quick or appear like an athlete, but I radiate happy energy. Energy I want to share with the world.

In the gym, I load weights on the bar, the clink bringing much satisfaction. I begin to pump myself up to a Beyoncé track, then I squat down, spine in line with my head and begin to deadlift. As I lift the weighted bar to my hips, I feel powerful. I see my reflection in the mirror. This girl can do anything. I drip beads of sweat, the endorphin high setting in, feelings of contentment spreading through me. My mind and body are released from any stress.

My days offer better structure with exercise in place. The small goals I achieve within my fitness encourage success in my work and personal life. This is time I have carved out for my body. It craves these workouts.

Fitness has always been important to me. If it's running, picking up/training weights, cycling, tennis, I'm all over it.

During a time I wasn't getting out of bed and leading a sedentary life, Shaun T's Insanity workout saved my life. To this day, fitness continues to save my life every day. Restoring my fitness gave me confidence and true happiness. Incorporating regular exercise and physical activity encourages strong muscles and bones. The benefits are endless. It improves respiratory and cardiovascular health, overall health, reduces your risk for type 2 diabetes, heart disease, and reduces your risk for some cancers. I have days where gentle yoga is enough. As long as I'm getting some movement each day, I'm content.

I found work at a local gym, teaching spin classes, and outside the gym began to build up my clients. My parents supported me one hundred percent, converting their garage into my gym. I only had two clients at the very beginning, and I now have forty-five. This wasn't easy. I hustled and still hustle hard. I reached out to people via Facebook, searching for people who were looking for personal trainers or wanting to get fit. I directly messaged them and had to sell myself and my skill set.

I needed to feel my bipolar wasn't a setback. I could still work and live a normal daily life.

When I trained my first client, I was nervous. I felt rusty in my knowledge, I felt I didn't look the part of having a strong fitness body - that perfect ripped body all people imagine personal trainers would have.

When I suggested to a client to keep track of his eating by using a food diary, he declined abruptly. I felt anxious and didn't want to upset him. He explained he had a stroke and often got confused, so he thought keeping a diary would be too strenuous. This meant I had to learn to adapt and be flexible as there were a lot of exercises he didn't like and therefore didn't do. I didn't give myself enough credit for being able to adapt to his needs, and we ended up achieving a lot in three months. Having bipolar made no difference. I didn't need to declare I needed medication, and it didn't hold me back.

I had felt vulnerable returning to work, and had doubts whether I could even help others when I couldn't even help myself at times. But this first client reassured my working abilities. Physically, he had lost a stone and a half, and he had started looking forward to our sessions. I felt disheartened when he took a break over Christmas and didn't return afterwards.

I realised then that I had done great work. Personal training is an investment in yourself, just like taking medication. Reaching goals can be amazing, but you then have to maintain it. His journey resembled my relationship with medication. Asking for help is a start, and reaching that small goal of feeling a bit better and taking the time as well as money to invest in myself is important. But quitting medication left me in the lurch. My first client quitting led him to regain the weight he had lost.

It is always okay if you still need help on your continuing journey.

I have grown a lot through my career. I am much more assertive, and make it clear that the exercises I give have a purpose. Even if the client doesn't like them, I now encourage them to give it a try anyway. One of my current clients, Samantha, told me I was too nice. I agreed at times I can be, but I have learnt it's knowing what approach to implement with each client. Some clients thrive off the 'no pain, no gain' chat, whereas others need a gentle approach and lots of friendly encouragement.

Over the months, I grew in confidence in my ability. I started out by charging just £15 a session but soon began charging more per session as my skills progressed. I still keep my prices affordable as I wish everyone to have access to help with their fitness, and this is how my client base has grown.

THE POWER OF MY CLIENTS

My clients are amazing - they have the ability to pull me up. I don't think they realise how much of an effect they have on me. I love my job and love who I work with.

One of my first and longest clients, Laura, dropped two clothes sizes, and two years later, I still train her today. A mum of two, she runs a business from her house. A truly inspiring fit mummy. Abs of steel and a heart of gold. She would always hear about my failed dates and friend dramas. I had been broken up with on one of the days I was training Laura, so I turned up, not wanting to cancel despite feeling very wobbly and teary. But training her made me feel better. She acknowledged my pain and reassured me I would feel better. I did. She smashed her workout as usual, and I felt inspired to train myself that day. She has that effect. We hugged at the end of our session. She fills me with light and gratitude, and my commitment to her prevented me from getting under the duvet covers and cancelling all clients and classes that day.

Karl, I have been training for over two years now, and his fitness journey has been inspiring. I now cycle alongside him, unable to keep up running with him. I always look forward to our chats, and we have that space to talk about a variety of topics, both deep and light. I feel like I'm not defined by my bipolar when I'm with clients like Karl, and it doesn't consume me. I vibrate with positive energy.

I helped Oliver with his marine fitness tests, and we now discuss history during our rest break between sets. History is important, and I am grateful to him. I feel us connecting when we discuss history, and my knowledge is forever increasing. I feel at ease and less anxious after I train Oliver.

Jade, one of my online clients, never fails to make me laugh. Her bubbly energy is infectious. I sometimes feel sluggish, mind not wanting to exercise, but as soon as I play the music, and see her face on my screen, I'm energised, ready for 25 minutes of intense exercise. I am excited for our journey to continue and for the goals we will reach together. She makes me accountable to show up and exercise, and supporting someone during their fitness journey is truly inspiring.

There is a sense of team and community with my clients. I have made many new connections, people have begun reaching out to me, and opportunities have started to present themselves. The days I feel low, seeing them makes me feel lighter. My clients and my personal workouts continue to save me every day. When I show up, and they show up for me, we put in the work, send out the positive energy to the universe, and good things happen to myself as well as them.

THIS GIRL CAN (SOMETIMES)

CHAPTER 18

CAT - but no meow

Bipolar can be triggered by trauma or life events. Sometimes, part of counselling involves addressing underlying concerns to get someone to a point where they can start to see a life worth living. I believe that counselling not only saved me but helped me actually manage my mental health in a healthy and positive way.

During my time with Dr Jean Rias, my healing process involved many different types of counselling, including Cognitive Behavioural Therapy (CBT) and Cognitive Analytical Therapy (CAT), where I became equipped with different strategies to manage my periods of lows or highs and began challenging or accepting difficult thoughts.

I started with CBT. Through these sessions, I monitored my mood via printed mood diary charts. This helped me see when I was most agitated and what I did before and after being agitated.

'I see you were agitated in the evening, what was going on for you here?' CBT counsellor Dan asked.

'Yes, I could not settle.'

'And what's the worst you feel could happen?'

'My head will explode.'

'It won't. Always remember this feeling will not last forever. It will pass.'

CBT was a great start to challenge my thoughts. It didn't delve deep, but it helped manage my anxiety.

In CBT, I learned how to monitor my mood. Essentially, how to check in with myself. My mood diary showed me if there were any triggers leading up to feeling low. I also kept track of what I was eating to see if certain foods impacted my energy levels.

In my psychotherapy sessions with Dr Jean Rias, we discussed at length the medication and the side effects. My concern about being on medication was the weight gain that might occur. She reassured me about the dosage I was on and always went through options with me. Having routine and structure is so important, it's one of the many things I do to keep me stable. I strive to do something that is the same every day and something that pushes me out of my comfort zone just slightly each day.

These days, I am not as rigid with my wake up time and bedtime, but having a balanced day does wonders for my mental health.

Dr Jean Rias sent me on a 12-session group CAT course, and this is where I met Lin, who ran the course. When she first told me, I imagined a group of us sat in a circle stroking cats. In reality, the therapy works by identifying any learned behaviours or beliefs from your past and investigating whether or not they are contributing to your current difficulties. CAT aims to show you how you can change such beliefs or behaviours, and help you focus on ways of making better choices in the future.

Through CAT therapy, we discussed the importance of kindness and the importance of being yourself. The days I felt low, I forgave myself. We can all have a critical negative voice telling us we aren't worthy or are not doing a very good job, and I'm now able to visualise hugging this critical voice, giving it love, compassion, and forgiving it.

CAT is an open and 'upfront' form of therapy, where the therapist shares their thinking with you explicitly. There are no hidden theories or secrets in CAT. The therapist is actively involved in treatment and will encourage you to be the same. This is something I found incredibly helpful in my recovery.

The therapist will work with you to identify your patterns, and they will understand the difficulties involved in change. We analysed our patterns and behaviours in great detail, and I discovered I had many patterns that I needed to reflect on, accept or challenge.

In the first session, we completed a questionnaire called 'The Psychotherapy File' which divides commonly experienced difficulties into Traps, Dilemmas, Snags, and Unstable States of Mind.

Traps - a trap is only a trap if you don't know about it...

Traps are things we cannot escape from. Certain kinds of thinking and acting result in a 'vicious circle' where, however hard we try, things seem to get worse instead of better. Trying to deal with feeling bad about ourselves, we think and act in ways that tend to confirm our badness. For example, my trap is as follows:

1. I believe I need to be in a relationship to feel okay
2. I am worried about being by myself
3. So, I don't try to be myself
4. With the result, I go from one relationship to the next
5. When one relationship ends, I don't want to be alone (back to 1)

Dilemmas – Nelly, I love you

Sat in my one to one with Lin, she said, 'We often act as we do, even when we are not completely happy with it, because the only other way we can imagine seems as bad or even worse.'

'I'm not sure if I follow.' I looked confused.

'False choices can be described as either/or, or, if/then dilemmas. We often don't realise that we see things like this, but we act as if these were the only possible choices.'

'So I choose to stay unhappy, as the other alternative seems bad or worse?'

'Yes,' Lin paused.

'I stayed with Jake, although I was unhappy, because being single, I felt would be even worse.'

'Okay, what's wrong with being single?' Lin maintained eye contact.

'Because then it confirms I'm unworthy of love,' I said, smiling sadly.

'Recognising this thought pattern is the first step to changing.'

I acknowledged this feeling of low worth and reflected on where it stemmed from. Then I came to the realisation that I had so much love within me, and I had so much love to give, and I should not fear love. It doesn't need to come from an external source - I needed to love myself first before I could really love another.

Snags - I snagged my own dress

'Snags are what is happening when we say, "I want to have a better life, or I want to change my behaviour but..."' Lin explained.

'Okay...' I responded.

'Sometimes, this comes from how we or our families talked to us when we were young. Comments from parents such as, "She was always the good child," or, "In our family we never..."'

'Can you give me an example?' I asked.

'Sometimes, the snags come from the important people in our lives not wanting us to change, or not able to cope with what our changing means to them,' Lin explained.

'No, I don't think I have experienced this,' I responded, thinking my parents and friends would never want to see me remain unwell or depressed.

'Okay, in other cases we seem to "arrange" to avoid pleasure or success, or if they come, we have to pay in some way, by depression, or by spoiling things. Often, this is because as children, we came to feel guilty if things went well for us, or felt that we were envied for good luck or success.'

'Ahh...Self-sabotage?'

'Yes,' Lin smiled.

'I do this, yes.'

'It's helpful to learn to recognise how this sort of pattern is stopping you getting on with your life. Only then can you learn to accept your right to a better life and begin to claim it.'

Together, we analysed my patterns.

My patterns:
1. I want to change the way I am
2. I make plans to lose weight
3. But why bother?
4. I don't deserve to be happy
5. Feeling frustrated and lonely (and going back to 1)

All these exercises are ways of helping to focus accurately on exactly what sorts of thinking or behaving contribute to things going wrong. Many of these function in conjunction with one another and sometimes fuel other behaviours, thoughts or cycles. I decided to focus on my vicious cycle of breakups leading to depression, and developed a self-awareness I hadn't ever experienced before.

At around session four or five, the therapist read to us a 'Reformulation Letter'. This is a written account of the understanding shared between yourself and the therapist about the problems that have brought you into therapy, how you have tried to cope with them, and what you are trying to change by coming into therapy.

My therapist, Lin, worked with me to map out my problem patterns on paper. This helped develop my capacity to think about myself and understand why I repeated patterns which caused me so much distress.

It became clear that I was not happy by myself. I needed to be in relationships to feel worthy and to have someone to do things with. In other words, I was unable to feel content with myself and my own thoughts.

Carrying out the work I was doing on myself outside of the sessions helped me build recognition of the patterns of relating, thinking, acting and feeling that I wanted to change. Lin's suggestion on ways of monitoring these patterns in between sessions, and looking out for these patterns happening within therapy itself, were extremely helpful. One of the strengths of CAT is that the letters and maps will help you to continue working after the regular therapy sessions have finished.

CAT recognises that finishing therapy can be difficult, especially if endings in your life have been difficult in the past. The last three or four sessions are used to think back over the course of therapy and the ending of the therapy relationship. The therapist will write a 'goodbye letter' and will invite you to do the same.

I checked in with Lin a few months after the counselling had finished and she was happy with my progress. I am grateful for this therapy and for meeting women from different walks of life. We supported each other as a group and helped each other. It was sad when it all came to an end.

THIS GIRL CAN (SOMETIMES)

CHAPTER 19

Diagnosis

When being given a diagnosis, it's tempting to hinge every experience and feeling you've ever had on the diagnosis. To an extent, it's a very natural thing to do, but you're still *you*. You still have your own feelings, thoughts, and your own voice and perception of your own life. Try not to adopt any illness as an identity. You are you. Whatever it may be, try to get to know yourself.

I now work with my bipolar rather than against it. In a strange way, we are a team, and pretending it doesn't exist never makes it go away. In fact, from past experience, ignoring my bipolar made it so much more difficult to control and added strains to relationships.

I tried coming off medication four times within three years, each time relapsing. Dr Jean Rias always supported my decision, and we would come up with coping strategies. It generally happens in the same way; I start off feeling okay but then fall into a depression meltdown. The last time I tried coming off was when I was 28 and seeing a guy who lived in Bristol.

We were dating for the summer and grew incredibly close. I had known him from sailing when I was younger, and we reconnected at a party in the summer.

I adored Liam. My heart wanted him, but I wasn't acting like myself, and I knew the future we held was unclear. When he called me his girlfriend, I felt hope for us. But he had me scattered in pieces, lighting me up like the brightest rays of sunshine he is, but then disappearing into his darkness, leaving me to wait. I felt lonely every second, like torture. There were many reasons to end the relationship, but I wanted him. I couldn't imagine a life without those breathless moments, but when he went radio silent, I knew we had little hope.

It was confusing, running on those highs of being together one moment, and then crashing to a low the next. A text from him would light up my day, and I went to great lengths to get him to notice me. I researched drum and bass artists, took interest in all his interests, and along the way lost part of myself. I became a shapeshifter, being whatever I thought he would like best.

Why did I do that? I jumped through hoops hoping to demonstrate just how special and unique I am, wanting him to stay with me.

I didn't stop and think whether it was a good situation for me, if we were happy, or even if my needs were being met. All I was focused on was being needed by him, instead of turning the focus to why I wanted to be with him.

When someone can't make up their mind, the price we pay trying to convince them that we're good enough is our self-esteem. The fact that we're going to all this effort proves to them that we actually aren't worthy, because if we were, we would know our own worth and I would have walked away a long time ago. I couldn't mend his soul.

I watched a documentary called Heal on Netflix. Inspired by people who had overcome disease and injuries through the power of the mind, I was convinced that my mind and body didn't need to be on medication anymore. I would heal naturally with sheer determination. But during the last weekend I spent with Liam, I became consumed with darkness and couldn't stop crying.

This might have been too much for him. He was battling his own demons, and I had been a crutch for him. I was a plaster, temporarily covering a deep wound, and when it was my turn to be wounded, he walked away.

I was heartbroken when he ended it with a phone call. His words were he 'didn't have the capacity to love me'. I took a few days out to grieve, something I should have done after my breakup from Jake, and what I discovered was life-changing. Perhaps for the first time in my life, I had determined my worth. I came to the realisation that I deserved more from Liam. When I gave myself love, priority and respect, other relationships blossomed. During this time, my friendship with Lexi flourished. Lexi is my strong, vibrant Canadian friend, who has helped see me through some very challenging times.

When I looked within and changed how I saw myself, the need for validation and relationships (friends and boyfriends) calmed down. This is still something I'm working on, and will continue to work on for the rest of my life. I now have that new sense of self-awareness I didn't have after the breakup with Jake. I am enough. You are enough.

I stopped wondering why Liam didn't want me. I started living my life again.

I went back on medication, and I felt better within a couple of days. I have now accepted that I may be on medication for the rest of my life.

THIS GIRL CAN (SOMETIMES)

CHAPTER 20

Sad endings

Three years had passed. I was 29, and Dr Jean Rias had some heartbreaking news.

'Good to see you looking well. How are you?' she asked, swivelling her chair to face me.

'Yes, good thanks, things have been going well…' I smiled, sitting down. The session was going well, and I concluded how I had been feeling better.

'Okay, I have some news,' Dr Jean Rias said towards the end of the session.

'Oh?'

'I will be leaving the unit.'

I froze mid-smile. 'You're changing jobs?' I asked slowly, trying to digest the news.

'Yes.'

I was so happy for her. She was moving on to new opportunities, yet I was in tears at the same time. She had been a stable force in my life for so long. She had seen me both at my very worst and in my current state, when I was doing okay. I had done so much growing because of her. She had met Dice, who came with me to understand more about my condition. This is a big deal for me — it was something my previous boyfriends never wanted to do, as any conversation regarding mental health made them feel uncomfortable.

I left the building, sat in my car and heaved heavy sobs. There's something about crying in my car, in the enclosed space which gives me a sense of security.

What would I do without her?

Dr Jean Rias said I would be seeing a new doctor.

I went to meet him the following week. As I sat opposite him, he gazed at his computer screen, and the room was silent. I looked at the ugly clock on the wall and fiddled with my necklace chain, waiting for him to start the conversation.

'From my understanding, you have been in remission for two years, no manic episode since, therefore, it's time we discharge you from the practice.' He said, finally looking at me.

The blow felt brutal. Someone had just pulled the rug from under my feet.

'I was hoping to come off medication…'

'You will never come off medication. You need to stay on it.'

I started to cry. He didn't even offer the box of tissues. I understood he was very much behaving as a doctor, but in my situation, I craved empathy, which I feel all therapists should give. Dr Jean Rias had set the bar too high.

The next few hours, I was trapped in a whirlwind of tears and dark emotions. I was grieving the relationship with Dr Jean Rias and was disappointed with her replacement. I spoke with my mum in tears. I spoke to my closest friends Fli and Lexi. I needed help. My poor flatmate must have thought I was suffering from a borderline personality disorder, going from tears to happy teaching a class online, then back to manic tears.

I was proactive - I looked into bipolar support groups and searched for counsellors who had experience with bipolar directly. The cheapest clinical doctor I could find cost £100 per hour. 'Money is not an issue,' my mum said. Gratitude and warmth flooded me. This is where my privilege comes into play. There are many people who aren't financially able to afford private counselling.

'But it is for me. That's two pounds a minute, I think I would be more stressed about that within the session.'

I opted for the lady who, although not a doctor, was a counsellor who had worked with clients with bipolar. I also joined a free bipolar support group called Bipolar UK.

The counsellor was fantastic. Straight to the point, she gave me the coping mechanisms I needed to get through my dark moments. I liked it when she said things like, 'I get you.' She tried to relate to me with language that I might use, and I appreciated that. When I had thoughts about cutting myself, she suggested running ice over my wrists, explaining the science behind the brain and why these feelings come and go. I scribbled a picture of what my darkness looked like, and then drew what I wanted it to look like. I learnt to engage with my five senses, and on the days I'm struggling, I keep my chess piece close to run my fingers over the edges.

The Bipolar UK support group consisted of twelve people, each seeming to be going through a hard time. I found myself drained after the session. I lay back on my sofa and closed my eyes. How resilient the group leader must be to run and listen to sessions like that. This group didn't work for me, but I could see the importance and value it had for the other participants.

I had to find the inner strength to find someone. Taking that first step of talking to someone, anyone, helped me come out of the whirlwind of darkness. For me, this was the hardest hurdle to overcome in recovery, but once I did, the light glowed again.

THIS GIRL CAN (SOMETIMES)

CHAPTER 21

I want to help people emotionally. I want to be a counsellor.

Whilst receiving my CAT counselling, I started my journey, age 27, to certify as a counsellor. Dr Jean Rias had inspired me, and without her, I would not have come out the other side post mental breakdown. We had achieved so much through the talking therapies, what if I could have the same impact on others? I wanted to help people with mental health issues as I knew first-hand how life-changing these talking therapies could be.

It turned out my former college nearby was running Counselling Level 1, 2 and 3 courses. When enrolling, I reassured myself I wasn't going backwards, and this would be a positive investment. The first class I remember thinking, '*Oh, no. What am I doing here? Will I be able to sit through the three hours and concentrate in this classroom?*' Luckily, my teacher for Level 1 and 2 was fantastic, with clear and organised teaching. We did a class icebreaker and then learnt the fundamentals of counselling. Throughout the weeks, we were introduced to roleplays and were taught the three key theories, person-centred, psychodynamic and CBT. It was the perfect introduction to counselling, and as a group, we felt bonded.

I had always thought it was only in London where you could meet a variety of people. But through my group counselling and courses, I met many strong, inspirational characters. We all passed with flying colours and progressed to Level 3.

The Level 3 teacher was not as organised as our first teacher, but I learned two rules out of the experience. Rule number one: Don't make suggestions to your clients. This made me laugh, as I knew of a counsellor who suggested I take long mindful walks as a solution to my anxiety, which felt condescending. Making suggestions in a counselling session can be dangerous, and can develop an unhealthy rapport. It turns out that a lot of the people studying with me had similar experiences with their counsellors. Rule number two: Less is more, and listening is key. As a class, we passed the exams, but through a lot of self-study.

We all went our separate ways, some continuing while others lost heart with the poor teaching. I was determined in my belief that I could help people and went on to a Level 4 course at another college. With my current counselling studies, I have explored much of my past and present values, beliefs and limitations. Developing a self-awareness, I started to see how I interact with others and how they interact with me. For example, after studying the PAC Triangle - standing for Parent, Adult, Child - I became aware if people were talking to me like a child, or if there was a mutual adult to adult conversation going on between us. Are they really listening? At a dinner gathering of ten friends, I could not believe how nobody seemed to be listening to each other. Conversations layered on top of each other, people responding without listening, giving advice and acting like the critical parent...if it weren't for my studies, I too wouldn't really be listening and speaking in a way that would be seen as mutual - adult to adult.

CHAPTER 22

I want to sleep, where's the off button?

Dear Sleep,

Let's be frank, we have a love-hate relationship, don't we? I have so much love and appreciation for you, and I need you. But sometimes you don't always need me.

You and I used to be such great friends. In primary school, in the car, on the boat, you would visit me on a regular basis.

At college and university, there were even some weekend mornings we spent together. I always felt recharged after seeing you.

There were times when you were too much, consuming my days. There were times we saw less of each other, but we still got along pretty well, didn't we? I wish I would have been more appreciative of you back in those days. I thought I was deprived of you, but I didn't know what the word deprivation meant.

Pre-breakdown, when I started seeing Ryan, I admit I was beginning to avoid you. We even lost touch for a while. I was busy socialising and going out in the evenings. I didn't prioritise you. I admit, having fun came between us.

During the breakdown, I cried for you to come, but you abandoned me. When you didn't come, I began to fear you. You took on this monster-like form.

Now, I miss you desperately. They say absence makes the heart grow fonder, dear friend, and you have indeed been way too absent lately. I find myself longing for you in the evenings.

Please, let's spend a night together, neutralise the relationship once again.

Just know, until that day when we can finally be together again completely, no tension, I'm always thinking of you, and I miss you.

We'll be together all the time again. I won't take you for granted. Remind me of these days so I can truly appreciate our time together.

Love always x

CHAPTER 23

"I love my husband, but it is nothing like a conversation with a woman that understands you. I grow so much from those conversations" - *Queen Beyoncé*

FRIENDSHIPS

At age 27, after my CAT therapy and CBT courses had ended, I was getting better and healthier: building on my new life, studying to be a counsellor, living with bipolar disorder. I was living at home, saving money, and had the support of my parents. I balanced my work and my social life. Now, equipped with different coping strategies, I could sense if I was dipping or if my high energy felt abnormal. I could track the majority of my relapses down to a shift in routine or a major life change.

Balance is important. I make time for family and friends, time for me to relax and have fun, and I aim for at least seven hours of sleep a night. However, there are days where I wake up feeling rough, and these are the days I fear as usually there are no triggers or warning signs, just a dark cloud hanging over me.

My mum once said to me, 'You don't need lots of friends, just a few that will be there when it counts.' Han, Fli, Jen, Lexi, Steph and Sophie make up my tribe. Han, I have known since college. Fli was someone I had invited out for a drink after a chance encounter. Jen never fails to make me cry with laughter, and Lexi, I met soon after Jen, and through our many walks together have gone deep in conversations. Steph is a loving mother hen. Sophie currently lives in Japan, and we have been friends for over ten years now. Tasha Eurich describes people with unique insights as unicorns in her work, *Insight*. These women, my tribe, are all unicorns.

In Eurich's work, she talks about the exercise of receiving feedback on yourself from people you trust. In the process of writing this book, the importance of knowing how people think of me became a necessity. Asking people for their unvarnished opinions of me gave me true insight into myself.

I decided to embark on an insight exercise for the present me. This exercise must not be taken lightly. The instructions are to carefully select the people to ask for constructive criticism and to ensure the conversation takes place when both participants are in a good space. I took a brave leap and asked Lexi how I came across. This exercise felt like a very brave thing to do as it highlights my flaws and negative attributes, which can be hard to swallow. Lexi wrote my feedback in a letter, and I wish to share how she introduced it.

Dearest Maria

This is my letter to you partaking in your exercise of self-improvement through receiving criticism from your friends. Please remember that you get to take what you want from this, if you disagree with it maybe burn it and let it go. This criticism is not yours to carry unless you reflect, something resonates, and you want to carry it forward. I am not any form of an ultimate truth, I am relaying my experience and observations with you, and they may be well off. I have tried to be as honest as possible and not hold back.

At first reading it, I felt fine, then I started crying. This is one of the hardest exercises I have ever done, and I'm a personal trainer. I had asked for the negative criticism because so many people fail to tell you what they really think. I was seeking an honest look into how my friend perceives me and what she thinks my weaknesses are. This was a part of my work of self-improvement. Although my opinion of myself should be the one that counts the most, having my close friend evaluate me gave me the opportunity to see through her eyes and fill in some blind spots. After receiving the letter, I found myself wanting to argue some of the points made, but that defeats the purpose of the exercise. It's my choice if I want to take things on, and, equally, I have the choice to dismiss them.

Things I already knew about myself:
- I don't practice my assertiveness enough
- I like to please people

New things I learnt through Lexi's letter:
- I filter my stories to portray the best version of myself
- I attach to labels strongly, e.g. Yoga Teacher, Personal Trainer
- I can be judgemental of other people's lifestyle choices
- I can push people into having conversations they are not ready for

I took some time to process the letter and came back to Lexi a couple of days later.

'I would like to clarify some things in your letter. Is that okay?' I said on the phone.

'Yes,' Lexi responded. I went on to explain the reasons behind why she must have felt I came across in particular ways. I acknowledged some of her points, but was honest about the things I disagreed with. Lexi listened and at no point interrupted me. When I had finished, she exclaimed, 'Well! I think this has been a productive exercise!' I agreed with her wholeheartedly. I feel a sharpness in my heart whenever I go back to the letter, but each time I read it, the sharpness becomes fainter. The fear of reading negative things about myself can be compelling, but this new awareness has unearthed a need to grow, weed out my flaws and flower. Having this experience, I move through the world differently, my awareness heightened and my eyes open.

I have experienced breakdowns of friendships, and when I asked Han what her insight was, she explained it well.

'You were lost back then, and you didn't know how to navigate yourself. So, therefore, others did not know how to navigate around you.'

'I was lost.' This was true.

Han went on to explain, 'You had tunnel vision and couldn't see from any other peoples' perspectives.'

'Han, what if all my friendships are destined to fail because of me?'

'You are a different person now; you can navigate yourself. The friends you have now know about your bipolar. Therefore, if the friendships you have now fail because it's too much, that's not a "you" issue, that is a "them" issue.'

I found it hard to maintain my friendships in London as I was living back home, and it was a 2-hour commute. Aside from Han, new female friendships had scarred me up until Fli. In school, the female group I was in always had some form of backchat and cattiness to it.

When I went to university, I met two girls, Sam and Vivian, who I thought were friends for life. But Sam could not cope with living with me even before my pre-bipolar diagnosis when I was suffering from an eating disorder. Then there was my American friend, Vivian, who after my mental breakdown, simply stopped replying and returning my calls. Vivian and I were incredibly close, having spent six weeks backpacking together. When she was going through a breakup of her own, I flew out to America to comfort her.

The cut off was brutal, and I felt hurt when she never explained why she cut me off. Five years on, I tried reaching out to her saying I was writing this book, and asking if she could give any closure. To my surprise, she responded. She felt I was acting selfishly and felt I was guilt-tripping her to talk to me during that period I was struggling. I wanted to rebut and explain my actions during that time and how incredibly sad I was to have lost her friendship, but instead, I thanked her, and to my surprise, she then apologised. I felt immediately lighter, and now we have a friendship again. During that time, she had just met a guy, and part of me felt she didn't want the 'unwell' me in her life, just like Jake. They only liked the 'fun' and 'happy' me. Instead, she told me she simply felt it was time for her to move on from our friendship at that time.

Friendships have broken down due to my illnesses, and for a long time, I believed I was the issue. But that changed when I met Fli.

Around Christmas time two years ago, Fli and I went for a drink. Sat opposite each other in the empty pub, we broke the silence and started to laugh as another sad Adele song began playing in the background.

I had been seeing her housemate George, now a good friend, and had clocked the keyboard in her flat, the pictures of Portugal filling me with curiosity. She seemed genuine whenever we had a conversation. I craved for a genuine female friend. As someone who had experienced rejection at school, she felt accepting. Having someone who felt authentic and grounded, I couldn't help but feel I wanted to be around her.

Talking to Fli was easy, and we planned a spontaneous trip to Portugal for our gals' version of Valentine's Day, *Galentine's Day,* where our ridiculous card drinking game solidified the friendship.

It wasn't long before we embarked on another trip together, this time to Bali. I found her genuine and caring. With those small feet of hers, she would trip up the mountains we climbed. 'Careful,' the local Bali tour guide would say after she tripped. This had me in stitches of laughter. I love her dearly. Up until meeting Fli, I struggled with meeting people, finding myself hanging out with my parents on a Friday night. I missed socialising with friends. Through Fli, I met new young people, which was difficult as Lymington has a very elderly population.

If ever I need help with a project, Fli is there to support me. Recently, she helped me write a song for Dice. She is an incredibly gifted musician, and she helped me create an extremely special moment. We share a love for *Tay* - Taylor Swift. I slid into her DMs a few years ago and am still waiting on hearing back, but nevertheless, I consider us close. There is nothing I enjoy more than when Fli gets her guitar out and plays a cover of one of Tay's classics. She's moving away this year. When she told me she had been offered a job, I gave her the biggest of smiles, clenching my teeth, holding back my tears - 'That's so great Fli!' If I looked like a bit of a psycho clown, she didn't say anything. I was so happy for her; she works very hard in her career, and she deserves this. She is a friend for life, and I will miss her. Numerous new friendships stemmed from meeting Fli: Alice, Steph, George...and all these people have been supportive of my mental health and have given me the space to talk. The support of these people is so important to me.

Although men and women can bond and form friendships, as females, we blossom on solid relationships with other females.

Such friendships can give females an outlet to share their problems, thoughts, experiences, feelings, and triumphs with those they feel that genuine, close bond with.

Women have been oppressed for many years, and the movement today of women building each other up is inspiring.

I cherish all the conversations I have with my tribe...the hilarious text messages I exchange with Jen, the inside jokes I have with Fli, the banter I have with Lexi, a general chit chat with a snuggle and cup of tea at Steph's. My emotional and mental strength comes from meaningful bonds with these strong females in my life.

I do believe with age we begin to surround ourselves with friends who have similar thoughts, beliefs, and actions.

An article published on the *New York Times* website states that women feel they can count on their friends to pull through for them, no matter what they are struggling with in their lives.

We can act as each other's emotional support system. We listen, give advice, hold each other, cry, and build each other's self-esteem. My tribe empowers me, and developing these strong and healthy female friendships is something I believe all females can benefit from.

Women can also be intuitive; for example, Lexi can sense in my voice if I'm holding back or if I'm about to share good news or bad news. I feel some women have a distinctive way of reading emotions and intuitively recognising what needs to be done before acting on it.

When my mum was diagnosed with cancer, she reached out to Lexi before telling me. Standing in the kitchen, I asked mum if something was wrong, feeling something had been off the past few days.

'The cancer has come back,' mum smiled bravely.

I could feel my world caving in, vision blurring from the tears as I attempted to process my worst nightmare.

'We will know how serious after some more test results.'

'Okay. You will be fine. You are strong. I need to get to a yoga class now, but I will call tomorrow,' I replied in a steady voice.

'Are you okay? I'm worried this may be triggering for you?' mum said.

'I'm fine. Honestly,' I smiled.

As I pulled out of the driveway, mum stood in the doorway looking on worriedly. I waved and smiled, but as soon as I turned the corner, I stopped the car and released heavy and painful sobs. Choking on my sobs, heart in agony, I wiped away the tears with the back of my hand, started the car and drove to the yoga class where I was meeting Lexi.

As soon as I saw her, she saw my eyes and embraced me.

'You know?' Lexi asked.

'I know.' I said.

'What do you need right now, we can skip yoga?' Lexi said.

'I want to do yoga.' I replied.

I spent the majority of the yoga class silently crying. Being instructed by someone else helped. I listened and carried out each pose slowly.

Sometimes, my tribe and I understand each other with no words. There are times I need validation which only my female friends can give. I needed Lexi's presence. She gave it without me having to ask.

I share some of my biggest vulnerabilities with my tribe. We share the honest truth with each other, we share intimate family details with each other, we discuss beauty products - for example, which vaginal hair removal cream is best - and we're honest with each other. If we think a guy is not attractive or an outfit isn't a win, we let each other know. Some more blunt than others - Steph...cough, cough. But above all, we share lasting memories with each other.

We rely on each other not only for a dress-shopping partner (or in my case swimsuits - a new obsession) but also to share those dark and raw moments, those moments which not all men are able to hear or know how to support.

I didn't tell my friends at first about having bipolar, but when the time felt right one night, around 2am, I had an unanticipated desire to write another blog revealing everything. I was 29, three years after being diagnosed. Restless in bed, it was like an itch I couldn't reach, an agitated energy which needed an outlet. I felt compelled to release this secret. Pulling my laptop out, you could only hear the rapid sound of me fiercely tapping on my keyboard, the glow of my screen illuminating my wide eyes in the darkness of the room. I was fixated. Words poured onto the page, and as I came to the end, calmness washed over me, my body grounded.

It was as if my mind, my body, and the bipolar were becoming aligned. I had slowly peeled back my hardened layers to expose a dewy warm lightness within me. I hit the share button to send to all my friends, my heartbeat quickened, my palms slightly clammy. I lay back in bed, 'Breathe,' I said out loud. I closed my eyes and eased into a peaceful sleep.

My friends' love and support the following day was blinding. Their words spread warmth through my entire body. I felt loved. How brave it can feel to be vulnerable.

If you are a female, no matter your age, treasure your friends who enrich your life, as they are the backbone of your support system.

THIS GIRL CAN (SOMETIMES)

CHAPTER 24

Yoga is life

When Fli and I were in Bali, we took a yoga class in Ubud. Ubud is yoga central, the streets full of people in yoga pants. It's the place all yogis travel to do their yoga teacher training. Not to sound cliché, but I completely fell in love with yoga in Ubud. I really found part of myself in Bali. Up until that point, yoga had seemed boring and a bit pointless.

We had some time to kill and had heard many tourists say how fantastic The Yoga Barn was.

'Well, we might as well give it a try, Fli?'

Tucked in the heart of downtown Ubud, we entered not knowing what to expect and wow, we found a tropical oasis. The vibrations hummed healing and renewal. The Yoga Barn's pace is intrinsically led by Balinese culture and is blessed by the Hindu and animistic traditions of Bali, embodying the healing medicine of Ubud.

Reading the information on the wall, 'The Yoga Barn invites all who enter the grounds to connect within and to experience life differently; it offers an opportunity for visitors to heal, to gather and grow in community; to connect to Self and to open up towards inner transformation.'

'Okay,' I said, giving a small eye roll to Fli. My mum is strongly into chi and energy, and I was open to it but hadn't directly experienced these energies.

We sat at the back in this yoga class. I slowly became connected with my breathing, and my movements began to feel fluid. The teacher was toned, tanned, and had a warm, fun energy surrounding him. In his loose vest and shorts, brownish hair tied back in the trending man bun, he led us through a great flow with clear instruction which kept me focused. He didn't need to raise his voice, yet his soothing and firm words reached the entire room. The space was open and earthy-smelling, with large door panels letting the natural light in. Despite feeling sticky in the humidity, skin moist with sweat, I was engaged in the present moment. Something I had never experienced completely. No technology to distract me, just my mind, body and mat. Contained was a special energy radiating from the space and teacher, an uplifting pulse that I felt throughout its wooden floors and the grounds beneath it. There was stillness, compassion, and inspiration in this space. "This teacher is fantastic, if only I could teach like that," I thought. The class was a big one, but even so, the teacher went around and acknowledged each person. From one simple adjustment, the pose I was in suddenly felt transformed. I felt empowered and wanted to know how he'd made me feel like this. I searched his eyes, my eyes wide with surprise, and he smiled back, knowing he had touched my soul. I decided there and then that this is something I wanted to invest in and grow in. The Yoga Barn is a world-class holistic destination with a heart and purpose, and I will forever hold gratitude to the teacher who started my yoga journey.

I came back to England and signed up for a yoga teacher training program in London. It wouldn't be the same experience as going to Bali or India to do my training, but I wanted to be certified so I could start teaching as soon as possible. I wanted to see if I could change lives through yoga and teach a practice which isn't so tough on the body. Personal training had served me well until that point, but there were times I had felt a particular client needed a slow session, a time to really connect the mind with the body.

CERTIFYING IN YOGA

The course ran over six weekends, and once certified, I immediately began teaching yoga at the gym where I was a spin instructor. I didn't feel I was getting into the groove of teaching. Up until then, I had only taught fitness classes where I had to be loud and motivational. I struggled to teach yoga as I hadn't connected with my own yoga practice since the class in Ubud. I am grateful for YouTube stars Adriane and Benji, who helped me develop my teaching practice. The flows and asanas (yoga poses) I chose were rigid, with no flow, and I did not connect with the people in the class. As a result, the class was not popular, and the manager felt best to close it. I was disheartened and felt sorry for myself. I allowed myself to be sad for a minute and then decided to reflect and identify what the key issues were. It came to me quickly. I needed to tune in with my personal practice.

One day, Lexi and I did yoga together outside. Lexi is a true yogi. She taught me that yoga did not always need to be a 60-minute perfect session. Sometimes it's just showing up on your mat, staying in Shavasana (lying down) for the entire practice. Lexi would even do a little dance mid-flow. It is important to not have expectations and just to show up as you are. That day, doing yoga together outside was such an incredible experience that I even wrote a poem about it afterwards. With no instruction, Lexi flowed into each movement, tuning into her breathing, listening to what her body wanted and then following it through with movements which served her, and her only. I was in awe - a true yogi goddess. I closed my eyes and turned inwards. Rigid at first, I started slowly flowing. I let go of the stress and the pressure of trying to look good in each pose. This is what yoga is about - feeling free. Here's the poem:

Yoga

Today with a dear friend
I did yoga outside
To work on some nice bends
New asanas I tried.
Feeling warmth from the sun
Felt the energy flow,
Motions fluid and fun
I perfected my Crow
Connecting with the breath
Calmness over the mind
Bend the body to the left
The practice wasn't timed
Setting the intention –
I do believe in me
Friend deserves a mention
I really felt more free

When I became more confident with my personal practice, I started a class called Home Yoga (teaching from my parents' open living room space, mum was thrilled). I became connected to the students and was able to guide a healthy practice.

THIS GIRL CAN (SOMETIMES)

For over two years now, I have been practising some yoga every day. Sometimes for only ten minutes. On weekends slightly longer. At the beginning, I would slot the practice into my day whenever convenient. In Downward Dog, my heels couldn't touch the ground, and my body was stiff, but I always felt better for it afterwards.

These days, I practice first thing in the morning for a minimum of ten minutes every day. Sometimes, on days I'm feeling low, my practice can consist of just me lying on my mat or staying in a child's pose. I play music sometimes, other times, I practice in silence. When I want inspiration, I follow YouTube videos. I am in love with my practice and yoga journey, and just the feeling of my mat grounds me. I wouldn't be able to manage having bipolar as well as I do without my yoga practice. The act of showing up for myself every day is spiritual. Where my job requires me to be there for people and motivate them in ways they need, this yoga practice every day is something I do solely for me, and it allows me the space to be with myself and reflect.

I built up a meditation practice. I started by using the popular meditation app, *Headspace*, but soon realising it was making me sleepy, I practised at the end of my yoga session. Just sitting on my mat, my chest lifting and falling for five minutes. It is never about blocking thoughts, but acknowledging thoughts and not holding onto them. Some days, I focussed on my breathing; other days, tears would be sliding down my face as I was feeling emotional turmoil. My mind, once so busy, was able to stream thoughts one by one.

I recommend meditation for every human on this planet. It allows one to stop, think, and breathe. Studies in Positive Psychology have demonstrated that those who meditate daily are better functioning humans in their routines. It is important to note that meditation is a personal experience and looks different for everyone. When I meditate, I sometimes enter a white, pure space and see another me sitting down. She is always relaxed.

The two versions of me start conversing.

'What's up? You seem a bit off today,' she says.

'I am,' I respond.

'Tell me about it.' And I would start offloading what's been on my mind. Sometimes, the other me can be dressed head to toe in designer clothes, other days she is dressed in black, smoking a cigarette. She finds me in my longer meditations and offers great comfort. She would always hug me goodbye and say, 'Love yourself, you're doing just fine.' I believe she represents my subconscious and is there to always offer me support.

Yoga and meditation go hand in hand and are friends with my bipolar, helping guide me to make better life decisions. This is why yoga is so important. It grounds me, and it gives my day intention, full of light and positivity.

CHAPTER 25

*Sparks fly: Get with me those green eyes, as the
lights go down...*

At 28, while I was travelling to London for my yoga teacher training, I would try to meet up with Tim, but something felt off. He had just launched his new business, and I put it down to him being busy. The time for us to be together wasn't right, because he needed to put all his time and energy into the business.

Around Christmas time, he asked if we could meet. I was excited to hear from him, so I put on a nice red dress and did my makeup. I was hoping I would end up staying the night at his, so packed a small bag to go straight to my yoga training the next day.

We met outside the tube station, and I greeted him with a kiss on the cheek like I always did. My spirit elevated, my smile full of anticipation, my heartbeat skipping. Things seemed okay, we were okay. We went to a hipster bar nearby, and both ordered water, laughing as we did so. Drinking wasn't really his thing, and I only drink when I feel like it.

Sat on the wooden benches, we were making small chit chat, but he seemed agitated. The space was crowded, and the music a little too loud. As we came to a silence, he took a sharp inhale and announced, 'I have something to tell you.'

'Okay...' My heart was pounding. Immediately, I thought he'd found someone else. It's not me. He didn't want me.

Tim then said 'This is hard for me. I have known since my early teens, but I have been in denial about it for a long time.'

He saw my confused looks.

He continued, 'I'm gay.'

I stared into those green eyes, completely shocked. The noise around us tuned out in my mind. This can't be.

He went on to explain he had struggled with it in his youth and thought that meeting me would help him 'become' straight. We had so much in common, and he respected me and cared for me. He loved me, but he wasn't in love with me. My heart was breaking. I looked down, eyes tearing up.

'Please say something.' Said Tim.

'But I love you,' and with that, I broke down sobbing.

'Let's get out of here,' he guided me out, tears streaming down my face.

'I'm going to go home.'

'No, please, let's talk, let me drive you home.'

We walked back to his flat in silence.

'Are you sure you are gay? Not just bisexual?'

'I'm sure.'

We got to his place, and there I cried some more.

Looking back, I made this about me. I did not stop to think how much stress and pain Tim must have been in all his life. Having to tell his parents. Having to carry such a heavy secret.

Driving me home, Tim looked at me.

'Are you okay?'

'I am.' But this was a lie.

When he dropped me back at the flat, I went inside and cried and cried. I called my mum.

'Well, that explains why he would never commit to you,' mum said, not seeming to understand why I was so upset.

'I wanted to spend my forever with Tim.'

'It's late, go to sleep,' mum responded.

I texted Jen, who immediately called me. She listened to my sobs with kindness and patience.

'I am so sorry. But of all the girls he thought he could make it work with, it was you.'

That made me feel better. He would never be with another girl.

I listened to *Sparks Fly* by Taylor Swift thirty times that day. The lyrics always made me think of Tim with his soul-searching green eyes.

I spoke to Tim's brother to help me process Tim's words, and he kindly expressed how he understood my hurt. I felt sad talking to him, but he helped me reflect on the situation and what Tim needed from me. I understood his parents weren't being supportive, and I needed Tim to know I would always support him.

Accepting that Tim and I weren't meant to be together was hard. But in my case, because of the bipolar, my thoughts transformed into darkness quickly.

I left London broken. For three days, I stayed in my room with the curtains closed. Some days, just lying on my yoga mat crying. In my depressive state, I would feel tired and sluggish. I found no joy in reading or watching things I would usually enjoy. I lacked confidence. I felt worthless. Worst of all, I felt suicidal. With eating, it would either be too much or too little, and I had no desire to exercise. I would avoid all my friends and family. However, mum would always come into my room, open the curtains, sit in the chair, and try to comfort me.

The contrast between my high and low moods worries me. When I feel good and have energy, I worry, is this part of the bipolar or is this me? Is this behaviour manic? When I feel low, the depression seems never-ending, everything in chrome, yearning to sleep and never wake up.

To help process this parting, I made collages of all the pictures I had of us. The memories brought back laughter and tears. Us playing Mario Kart in the arcade, us working out, us dressed up for dinner. I messaged these collages with the words, 'You will always have my love and support, but I worry, Tim. What if I never meet anyone as great as you?'

Tim instantly responded with this message - 'I have absolutely no concern about that whatsoever. Zero. You are articulate, funny, intelligent and very attractive. And EURASIAN. You deserve a lot and you'll get it.'

Tim and I weren't meant to be, but he will forever be my friend, and he will forever have a small piece of my heart. And he was right - I did find someone else. I fell in love with Dice, and he is by far my greatest love.

CHAPTER 26

You always gain by giving love

Love. It's a word that can come naturally, be overused or avoided. Many people, philosophers, neuroscientists and clinicians have explored and talked about love. We can use this word for so many emotions.

Love has been transformative to my recovery. Reading my diaries, I can see that I have experienced a range of different loves. The Greeks distinguished different types of love and have a Greek word for all of them. I understand there are many sources and languages that define many other kinds of love, but these are the four key types that resonate with me.

EROS: EROTIC, PASSIONATE LOVE

Age 27

Dear Diary

I haven't heard from Liam. He's at a music festival, and I'm trying to be the cool and calm girlfriend, but I know his ex-girlfriend is there. On my birthday we spent the night on the boat, bodies entwined, souls connected. I resented the morning light as I wanted this night to last forever. He had been unsure if he would be able to make it down as he had been feeling low, but he made it, and it was magic.

When we are apart, my mind is consumed with Liam. I'm agitated, checking my phone, fingers burning to press the call button to him...Is this healthy? I've never felt this kind of love before.

Eros is a passionate love. It's often all about need. My love for Liam was addictive. It caused great joy and great pain. This type of love isn't always good for you, and in my case, it wasn't sustainable. I needed this kind of love to come to the realisation his love wasn't good for my mental health, and what I needed to avoid when I was next ready for a new relationship.

PHILIA: LOVE OF FRIENDS AND EQUALS

Age 29

Dear Diary

As Dice was reading his book, I fell asleep in his arms. Warmth, safety and contentment radiated through me. This moment was magical, my love for Dice is a steady flow. No words needed to be exchanged for his love glistened. Some people wait a lifetime for a moment like this.

Love, let what is beautiful be beautiful. It can be the love between lovers when they've been together for a long time, not driven by passion. Let this love with Dice forever speak to me, even if it's a memory. His love has provided support to my bipolar, my ups and downs. The steadiness of Dice's love grounds me in a way I thought not possible. I find it hard sometimes to fully notice the love and beauty in real-time, but when I reflect, like sitting having breakfast together, a real love was present, and when he leaves Lymington, my soul will still know how to hold onto this love. I trust there will be more to come.

Philia is the accepting love of a good friendship, and it's this love that's good for you. For me, this love lowers my stress and any physical pain. I fill myself with more positive emotions, and knowing I have Dice as a partner in my journey strengthens my ability to manage my bipolar. All of these are positive consequences of philia love; loving friendships make us more resilient when hard times come.

STORGE: LOVE LIKE A PARENT FOR A CHILD

Age 11

Dear Diary

I met Vita today. She is a stocky baby and had many folding rolls. As mum was driving me to visit, I stared out of the car window in a grump. I wanted to continue to be GMK's favourite, but now she has her own baby, where does this leave me? I knew I was thinking selfishly, but I like feeling special. Walking through the door, GMK embraced me, kissing me twice on the cheeks. She was glowing. I looked past her and saw the round baby. I walked over slowly, ready to say hi and bye, but seeing Vita's face, my heart melted. Her chunky hand wrapped around my finger. She gurgled and smiled. 'Wow,' I thought.

I understand this is the kind of love parents have for children, but I felt connected to Vita through my love for GMK. I wanted to protect her, and this love changed me. It's described as the most natural of loves. I would do anything to ensure Vita is okay. When I'm feeling suicidal, I think of how Vita would react if she had discovered I'd chosen to end my life without saying goodbye to her. This inflicts deep sorrow. I would never get to witness all the great things she will do with her life. I want to be her role model. I want to be here in case she ever needs me.

AGAPE: LOVE FOR HUMANKIND

Age 29

Dear Diary

George Floyd is dead, and there are protests worldwide. I need to take action. This can't continue. There are so many issues that need to be addressed. Our next World Stages Now drama performance will be about the Black Lives Matter movement. I will apply for funding, our performance will address key issues and bring awareness to audiences about why we need to talk about this.

This is a love bigger than just me, my family and friendship circle. A love for all. This love fuels me to dream big and spread love to those vulnerable. It is an unconditional love I aspire to.

PHILAUTIA: LOVE FOR SELF

Age 21 - Living in Japan

Dear Diary

I feel royally messed up. I have been avoiding my grandfather, and my actions are cruel. This is not me. I love my ojiichan (grandfather), and it is not in my nature to behave this way. I'm feeling unwell. My body feels weak. I don't have the energy to sit and talk with him. But how can I forgive myself for treating him this way?

It's the love that is given, whether or not it's returned. It's love without any self-benefit. In the Buddhist tradition, it is the central foundation of loving - kindness for all humankind. This kind of love is important in the process of forgiveness.

I love myself, and my *ojiichan* loves me, and I need to forgive myself. I know my *ojiichan* forgives me. Forgiveness is important, because from this experience the inability to forgive is associated with resentment and the anger towards the self, and the impact on my body was damaging. I understand this love is challenging, but it sets the foundation for happiness and contentment. When I feel suicidal, I have learnt to forgive myself. When I don't exercise, when I overeat, I try my best to forgive myself and love myself.

THIS GIRL CAN (SOMETIMES)

CHAPTER 27

"Forgiveness says you are given another chance to make a new beginning" - Desmond Tutu

Life was good. I had moved out of my parents' house, feeling at 28 it was definitely time to start being independent again. My counselling course was going well, my yoga teaching was developing and growing, and I even started teaching yoga to young children at a school and had a yoga class for the elderly. I have grand visions of spreading the power of yoga to all ages. I had a wide clientele I personal-trained, and I taught Japanese on the side. I purchased a flat near my parents' house and moved out. I felt strong and independent.

At this point, I was still seeing Dr Jean Rias once every few months to check in with my medication and any big life updates. Sat in the mint green chair opposite Dr Jean Rias, she faced me, hands clasped on her lap, warm smile, body language neutral. She opened the conversation.

'What would you like to talk about today?'

'I'm worried about moving out.' She noticed me wringing my wrists.

'Okay, can you cook?'

'Yes.' I said with a nod.

'Do you have a support network in place?'

'Yes.' I said with another definite nod.

'Then I see no reason why you can't do this. Remember, you have done it before during your time in London, and you can do it again.'

In her room, I brought in my life experience, my own personal circumstance (family, work, interests), and how I was feeling. Dr Jean Rias brought years of valuable knowledge, study, and experience from treating others. We worked together. Respected each other. She would sometimes ask tough questions, and I sometimes asked her tough questions. I was doing well, and I seemed stable, but this changed.

SASKIA

A friend of mine moved into my newly purchased flat. My first impression of Saskia was that she was grounded, and I felt we had a lot of common interests. She was into reiki and healing people. She had travelled a lot. Beautiful blonde hair framing her elfish face, cool nose stud, I liked her. We had talked about moving in together, and after her relationship came to an abrupt end, the natural course was for her to move into my spare room. She was a friend in need, and I had a place for her to stay.

She had big plans to move abroad, and I became worried I would have a vacant room and no way to pay my mortgage. There were rising tensions between us, and living together was becoming rocky. Not the smooth transition I had anticipated. I needed to know what her plans were so I could focus on getting someone in the room after she left. When I messaged her asking what her plan was, things escalated quickly, going from bad to worse before she blocked me from contacting her.

After she blocked me, I was upset and disappointed with how things had turned out. It was for the best she moved out before the friendship soured even more. We chatted face to face in the morning. I found the confrontation traumatic. My reaction was slow, and all I could do was listen. I broke down crying afterwards. Her behaviour felt triggering, reminding me of my PR manager back in London. I felt extremely on edge and anxious. I replayed the conversation.

'Saskia, bills have gone up with you having the heating on. Can you contribute any more? Don't you think it's best you move out?'

'No, I have nowhere to go, if you kick me out, where will I go? You have been so kind letting me stay, but the room is not worth any more than what I pay.'

'Okay, so when will you be moving out?'

'I don't know!' she was shouting at this stage, and I remained silent. 'You will be the first to know when I figure my life out. I've been going through a really tough time.' We stared at each other. I didn't know how to respond.

In any conflict, it is never a good move to attack the individual, and I felt attacked. So, Saskia refused to move out. I moved back to my parents' for the remaining three weeks, and I let my room to my new tenant, Ingrid. When Saskia left, Ingrid moved into her room, and I moved back in.

After Saskia had moved away, she got in touch half a year later. She apologised for how she had behaved and said she was in a bad space mentally, which resulted in her taking out her frustrations on me. Time allowed us to feel less raw. Forgiveness is everything where it is genuine. 'Water under the bridge,' I responded. With time, great reflection and insights can happen, and a valuable lesson I have learnt is it is never the argument that matters, but the ability to rebuild and repair.

Saskia leaving meant that I met Ingrid. I am a strong believer that everything happens for a reason.

When I first met Ingrid, she was carrying a yoga mat. She told me she was training to be a counsellor at the same college I had completed my Level 3 training. She had just gone through a breakup, and she was letting herself be vulnerable sharing her story with me. She took a moment to breathe and swallow her tears down. I felt my eyes water. When she left, it felt natural to hug. I felt warm. This was a good feeling. Oh, how brave it is to be vulnerable.

We live together in harmony, and I am forever grateful she came into my life. A bad day can quickly be turned around receiving a smile from Ingrid.

CHAPTER 28

GMK - AKA, the real superwoman

I mentioned my godmother earlier. I know her as GMK, Godmother Kate. She deserves a chapter just about her as she is someone I admire and love deeply. She was there during my breakdown, and she helped with my recovery when I came out of the institute.

I have learnt to do things for the me that's growing. I'm tired of making myself small and unnoticeable. I deserve to take up space and stay open, vulnerable and brave. I want to live a life full of love, just like GMK lives her life. GMK is such a powerful source of light and energy and shows me I can have a fulfilling career and a loving family.

GMK is the invisible crutch for me. She acts in a similar way as my chess piece...I don't always need it on me, but knowing it's there, she's there, is grounding.

She took the role very seriously from a young age when my parents asked her to be my godmother. GMK had just turned 16. As I grew older, she would take me on shopping trips, and invite me over to the farm in my hometown for dinner; and when she asked me to be a bridesmaid at her wedding, she laughed when I refused to wear the dress she had designed. I was very much a tomboy back then and refused to wear a dress, so I wore a Japanese kimono instead. GMK is just extremely cool. When she told me she was pregnant, I wasn't over the moon. I liked being her goddaughter, and I felt jealous. That was until I met my godsister Vita, and wow, she was a very sturdy baby. She looked just like her grandfather, Jonathon, and as she grows up, I see more and more of my godmother within her. I'm so happy to be part of their family. GMK has been such a stable role model and has impacted my journey navigating through having bipolar. I know I can always turn to her, and she will carve time out of her busy schedule to see me.

A dinner I will never forget with my GMK, was when I told her about starting up my business with Saturn, my business relationship, and new boyfriend Jake. She asked me, 'Is your business partner putting in the work? Are you yourself bulletproof so that you could live with or without a boyfriend? You need to be happy with yourself, never give up your interests, and be the one able to support yourself financially.'

Those words have never left me. They are the same words I said to Vita when she was old enough to understand them. George, her father, had agreed with me when I declared once at one of the dinners at the farm, 'Never waste your time with silly schoolboys, Vita. Focus on you.'

CHAPTER 29

My gratitude letter to GMK

Dear GMK

The day you got married, I was dazzled by your beauty and love.

I have always been blessed to have you as my role model to look up to, with your love and wisdom it gave me the ability to spread my wings and fly off into the world on my own to find myself. 'The world is your oyster,' as your husband once told me.

I can always turn to you.

I always want to make you proud.

After we completed the Round the Island Race, I turned to you and said, 'I love you,' and you smiled back and said, 'I love you, too'. I am overwhelmed by this love.

I was never told who to be, or what to do. I was guided through life, and when it was finally time to fly, I was ready, and I only have you and my family to thank for that.

Love

Your Goddaughter

THIS GIRL CAN (SOMETIMES)

CHAPTER 30

My lucky Dice

Dice and I met in university when I was 20 years old. We met at Waseda University in Japan and became close. With his bleach-blond hair and passion for football, I thought he was a nice guy. He wanted to date back then, but I was already in a long-distance relationship with James, who I had met in my first year of university in London.

Dice and I managed to stay in touch over the years. He had heard about many of my failed dates and boy troubles, and I would listen to his struggles with his on/off Japanese girlfriend.

After another failed relationship and knowing he had broken up with his girlfriend for good, I messaged him - 'Fancy a rebound weekend getaway?' The timing would be perfect as he would be in Amsterdam for work. 'Sounds fun. Let's do it,' he responded.

He met me at the airport terminal, and he was casually leaning over his luggage, book in hand, wearing a cream cardi, sleeves rolled. When had he got so tall and attractive? I spotted him before he spotted me, and I felt butterflies. I didn't remember him being this cool, but as soon as we made eye contact and hugged, I knew he was still the same guy I had met all those years ago.

On the train ride from the airport, we unpacked everything. My failed relationships, his nightmare breakup, where it had gone wrong, and now what we were looking for in the next relationship. To my surprise, I discovered we had similar values. We both had the desire for our children to be brought up bilingual. I want my children to value their Japanese inheritance and appreciate the language and the culture, and he feels the same. I had tried to hide my Japanese heritage growing up, and I don't wish that for my children. I had always felt it would be easier if I had a partner who knew some Japanese to help bring up children with a second language.

We spent an amazing three days exploring the city on foot. Eating out, drinking beer and playing pool. Amsterdam is one of the greatest small cities in the world. From Amsterdam canals to world-famous Amsterdam museums and historical sights, it is one of the most romantic and beautiful cities in Europe. A dream came true for me, as I saw the famous sunflower painting in the Van Gogh museum. We walked by Anne Frank's house, something I had always dreamed of seeing. All the winding canals and cute bridges led to new sights and places. We spent one morning at an adorable pancake house, and he asked the waiter to take our picture. This would be our first picture taken together there.

Growing up, I felt previous boyfriends had never asked to have pictures taken together, and it had led me to feel they didn't want to be seen with me. Looking at the root of it, I was concerned because I thought they felt embarrassed to be with me. For him to take the initiative of wanting a photo made me feel I wasn't embarrassing to be seen with. Given the mental health issues I have endured in my life, I sometimes to this day find things triggering and difficult to navigate. This moment, small as it was, had a huge impact on me as I knew he *wanted* to be there with me.

The buildings and architecture were breath-taking. Cobbled roads, new and old buildings blending into each other, always looking both ways before crossing to ensure we wouldn't be hit by one of the many cyclists...The rebound fun ended up not being the focus of the trip anymore.

He came back to my hometown for a few days after his Amsterdam business trip. At that point, I thought the relationship wouldn't develop any further, but we ended up speaking every day after he left. I was still dating other people, albeit unsuccessfully. Dice asked me to be his girlfriend a few weeks after Amsterdam, but with him living in Japan, I couldn't see how the relationship would work.

'Tell me the plan, how will this work?' I said on the phone.

'I haven't got that far...' Dice replied.

'I don't want to do long distance. It won't work.'

So I continued dating, one shocker after another. There was Steffan who offered no intellectual conversation and somehow paid for no dinners, even the one on Valentines' Day. My friends couldn't believe me when I simply messaged him, 'Thank you. Next!'

Oli was different. He had a beautiful dog called Tala, and he was genuine and caring, but Tala would always be his number one and something didn't quite match up.

Then there was the Asian doctor, Greg, who was into some weird things. I remember he asked Alexa to play *The Weeknd* and Dice's favourite song, *Starboy,* came on, and I felt my heart pang in sadness that he wasn't the one here instead.

There were so many dates, and it was fun, but with each guy, Dice was in my mind and in my heart.

Dice then informed me he was quitting his corporate job and moving to Spain. I was beyond excited - he would only be a 2-hour flight away. I did so much journaling and had many confused conversations with my girl tribe.

Cons

- He plays a lot of poker

Pros

- He makes money through poker
- He wears nice jumpers
- I can be my complete goofy self around him
- Since Amsterdam, all my dates have been unsuccessful as Dice is always in the back of my mind
- I love him. I love him. I love him.

On May 20th, 2019, I asked him to be my boyfriend. His kindness and love overwhelmed me. Our relationship is far from lovely and perfect. No relationship can be roses and unicorns all the time. It can be tough. We went for over three months without seeing each other, and I struggled. I managed to maintain a busy and social work/life balance, but I missed him. In our long-distance relationship, particularly when there are long periods where we don't see each other, I need a lot of clear communication. There were times we misunderstood each other's messages and annoyed each other. I once even cried on the phone to him not to bother coming to England…yet we got through it. We have had fighting matches that could have been a cliffhanger scene on EastEnders. We have definitely seen each other's worst sides, but have always found ways to repair and come out better on the other side.

I like to think I am now independent. I have learnt and reflected on my past failed relationships, where I was overly dependent on my partner. I want Dice's love and his intimacy, but I want to keep the freedom my career brings. I think Dice loves my earthiness, and I love our shared humour and his beautiful laugh.

I feel we support each other in all our ambitions and goals. He supports me in my big life-changing career goals, but he also challenges me often on the little things. For example, he called me out once for trying to order a salad.

'Why don't you just make it yourself? You have all the ingredients...' he said as I was scrolling takeout delivery services.

'I want to treat myself.'

At first, I was in a huff but ended up making one of the best salads ever at home.

Mental health should be talked about. It can be a hard topic, but if you're experiencing something, having someone to share it with can be life-changing. Without Dice, there would have been some very lonely and hard times.

Dice will stay on the phone with me on the nights I can't fall asleep. Without Dice, my periods of darkness would be drawn out much longer. I cried one night, insisting I needed to go back to my parents, and he sat with me on the floor and held me until I stopped crying. He came with me to meet Dr Jean Rias and asked questions. He doesn't always understand what I'm feeling, but he sits with me through any distress or pain. I think this is so rare, and reflecting on it, I can't help but feel overwhelmed with gratitude for his enduring love and bravery.

Dice holds my space, he holds my hand and doesn't try to fix me when I'm in a negative spiral. There is no judgement or fear of abandonment. We choose to talk rather than walk away.

It is important that when love appears in your life, no matter what part of your journey you are on, you let it happen. I love Dice, and leaning into this love and relationship has changed me for the better. I never want to stop loving and allowing myself to be loved. We have intertwined our souls so together we can create a life that gets a little better each day.

We walk side by side through this life supporting and loving each other as partners and teammates, and I cherish that.

CHAPTER 31

World Stages Now - theatre that empowers and brings communities together

World Stages Now is a Southampton-based organisation that provides a space for asylum seekers and refugees to collectively and creatively address issues of migration through drama and performance. I have always loved drama, and have been a member of this group for many years. We devise pieces of theatre together that encourage vital skills in listening, sharing and inclusion in order to translate ideas into an art form that reflects and articulates the needs of our community.

'Apathy is oppression. We are the problem, not speaking up is the problem.' - Lexi Dutnall

I can't sit by and do nothing.

I feel I'm making a difference in my own small way, and being part of this group offers new insight and allows me to see the bigger picture. They pull me out of the bipolar and make me feel accepted and like I belong. These Black women are strong, independent, loving and protective. The majority of the performers, writers, directors, musicians and dancers have been on an incredibly difficult journey seeking asylum. I believe through our performances, we are making a small difference, tackling important issues such as race, inclusion and history. By inviting our audiences to participate, through dialogue, discussion and active debate, we are educating our audience.

THIS GIRL CAN (SOMETIMES)

Since 2013, we have created and performed several pieces of original theatre - in particular for Refugee Week - exploring issues that are personal whilst also celebrating the national theme.

During the time I was vulnerable and first managing my bipolar, these women welcomed me with no questions and open arms. Walking into every rehearsal, no matter what was troubling me would ease as soon as I saw their loving smiles. I have grown with these women. I have seen their joy and their pains as they have seen mine.

The 2020 Black Lives Matter movement fired me up. There is me before this movement and me after. The death of George Floyd was the catalyst for a movement of protests and calls to action across the world. This movement exposed and opened my eyes to these injustices of unfairness. From this movement, I felt it was my obligation to educate myself on what it actually means to be Black in the UK. I have been naive in thinking that the disparities and injustices that my friends in World Stages Now experience are smaller and less obvious than in reality.

A lot of these women have experienced heavy trauma, and it hurts my heart to think that some of them are denied opportunities to address their health because of their race. I now feel it is my obligation to stand by them, listen to their stories and help them create their path to justice. Of course, all lives matter, and to all the white readers, your pain is important, real and hard. However, the way in which Black people walk through the world is something I will never experience, and the way in which they are institutionally cast aside is exclusive. I acknowledge that the pain they feel is a level of pain I will never experience. I want to make it my mission to empathise and address this pain.

It was time to do my research and have those hard chats with clients and friends.

I discovered racial disparities still exist even after controlling factors such as income, insurance status, age, and symptom presentation in mental health.

On their website, the organisation BlackLiveMatters.com explains some of the key barriers, including:

Different cultural perceptions about mental illness, help-seeking behaviours and well-being

This made me realise that when receiving or giving counselling, race may be a very important factor to consider, which led me to further reading. It is more than appropriate to address the difference in race in the first session if it will help build an understanding. Never will I state to my future clients that I understand their issues. Everyone experiences things differently.

Racism and discrimination

To this day, people are treated differently because of their race.

Greater vulnerability to being uninsured, access barriers, and communication barriers

Why should one's race affect their credibility to be insured?

Fear and mistrust of treatment

I see it within my Black friends. The fear behind their eyes from scarring past experiences.

I have experienced some hardships in my life, but I cannot imagine having to experience this not having had access to the resources I did. Having distanced myself from my Japanese heritage growing up with fear of being different, I am familiar with this feeling of staying quiet. There are some people who have chosen to not acknowledge racism, and this isn't right.

CHAPTER 32

Dear White Readers

In my experience with bipolar, I was fortunate to have a family support system and support from my doctor and the NHS. My race was not an issue. Yes, I had negative encounters with bipolar from others, but not because of the colour of my skin.

It is time to feel uncomfortable. The pervasiveness of mental illness stigma is often higher in ethnic minority communities, and this is mainly because of prejudice and discrimination towards ethnic minorities from our - your - society.

Did you know an overwhelming majority of people from Black, Asian and Minority Ethnic (BAME) backgrounds in the UK living with mental health problems face regular discrimination because of their illness?

The anti-stigma organisation, Time to Change, conducted a survey exclusively of people from BAME groups, and 93% said they had experienced discrimination in everyday life due to their mental health difficulties.

Areas of life where discrimination was commonly included:

- Places of employment
- In communities
- Within families
- And, during contact with mental health services.

Some groups, such as young Black men, are much more likely than the wider population to be subject to sectioning under the Mental Health Act, to be held in seclusion in mental health units, to be physically restrained (in some instances causing death), and to face discrimination due to what campaigners have argued are misguided perceptions of 'dangerousness' or propensity to violence.

Campaigners have consistently argued that there is institutional racism within mental health services, leading to poorer outcomes for numerous BAME patients...

Can you understand why this fires me up?

However, because I doubt myself and don't want to offend anyone, I stop speaking up.

Attitudes towards people with mental health problems can be shocking. I believe a better understanding within the system of people from different cultural backgrounds is a necessity. Understanding the degree of discrimination, and its various forms, is vital, and attitudes both within services and in wider society need to change.

I went to a Black Lives Matter protest alone after little discussion with my friends and family, not wanting any hard conversations. I feel I am now faced with the choice of staying quiet or speaking up with the risk of alienating my friends, clients and family. But I don't want to stay polite or quiet anymore. Let's talk, let's read, and let's educate ourselves.

BAME having equality in the mental health services is important to me. When I begin counselling, the issue of race will be an open conversation.

So, if you are a reader afraid to speak up because of your fear of judgement, work on letting that go. We will all get it wrong. More than ever, this is the time to educate, listen, read, and talk about key racial and mental health issues.

CHAPTER 33

Blind-sided by darkness

I wake up, I practice my yoga and meditate. I start my working day, and all seems well. I sit down with a green tea in hand for a short break and then with little warning it slams into me, this huge weight full of darkness, consuming my body and mind.

I stand, I pace, I want to shake this feeling off. Fear begins creeping in, knowing my mind is starting to travel down a dangerous path. My chest becomes tight, the thud of my heart is alarmingly loud. 'Breathe,' I say out loud. Tears start streaming down my face. I try to focus on my breathing, but it's not enough. Tears turn into waterfalls, face crumpling, body shuddering, I bury my head into my hands. I despise myself. The hatred is strong and poisons my mind.

'Make it stop, make it stop.'

'Make what stop?' I argue with myself.

'I can't see the light.'

'You have food, water, shelter. You have wonderful family, friends, and a loving dog. You have a functioning, strong body. You should be grateful. Why are you not grateful?'

But in that moment, none of it matters. Collapsing onto the floor, hugging my knees and gasping for air, all I want to do is put a bullet in my head.

THIS GIRL CAN (SOMETIMES)

CHAPTER 34

The importance of talking about suicidal feelings

I break it down to having good hours and bad hours. I especially struggle during the evening, sometimes feeling my chest tighten, my mind anxious. Something that still lingers post-bipolar diagnosis. There was a time I was unable to sit with my thoughts, but I know this is not the issue anymore.

As I said earlier in the book, I worry about the days I wake up feeling rough. Mind heavy, crying throughout the day, with the frustration of there being nothing to be sad about. I have to keep telling myself: this is not me, this is just the bipolar.

Having suicidal thoughts is a common depressive symptom of bipolar disorder. Without treatment or talking about it, these thoughts could get stronger. The risk of suicide for people with bipolar disorder is fifteen to twenty times greater than the general population. Studies have also shown that as many as half of all people with bipolar disorder attempt suicide at least once.

I struggled with letting my friends know when I was feeling suicidal. So Jen came up with a code word. If any of the girls posted 'bleacher' in the all-girl messaging group, this would be a code red. We would drop everything to check if that person was okay. Building a circle of support is so important. Friends, family, professionals, community resources...all can help. I have learnt how important it is to reach out to others when I am unwell, even when I don't feel like being around others. Going through episodes alone has had some disastrous consequences in the past.

If I killed myself, it would not only destroy my family; my friends would be heartbroken. That is something I try to hold onto in my darkest times.

I am grateful for the days where I wake up full of energy and ready to take on the day. I never fail to do my morning ritual of coffee, yoga and meditation, and taking medication with lemon water. My routine is in check, and on those days I am fun, positive and able to support my friends in any way they need me to.

I have learnt that a true friendship consists of balance. Balanced conversations are essential for a fulfilling friendship, and both must feel heard. Both people must have a chance to share information and stories. When conversations focus solely on one person, the other will become bored or hurt over time. Conversations should go back and forth in order to feel fair and satisfying, and above all, it is important to listen to your friends, give them your full attention.

The days I'm well, I can message my friends saying, 'I am feeling good, if you need any support or a chat, here to listen.' The times I'm struggling, I will message, 'I am working through some things, I will be in touch.' I have found when I am not in a good place, it's hard to help my friends.

CHAPTER 35

Binge eating mania

I have many people to be thankful for, but I wouldn't be where I am without my mum.

Mum is a legendary hero. She is my rock. Thinking about living a life she's not in panics me. Having gone through her own battles, she is strong and wise. She even flew across the world to support me during my year abroad in Japan when I was battling a binge eating disorder.

This was all pre-bipolar diagnosis, back when I was at Waseda University in Tokyo. It started with me wanting to conform to Japanese body type standards and taking a passing comment that I was fat to heart. I started watching and restricting what I ate, and I dropped weight to the point where my body went into starvation mode.

I began eating my lunch by myself, tired of comments being made on how little I was eating, or why had I lost weight. The lowest point was eating my lunch in the bathroom. I didn't want to be seen by others.

My body was breaking down electrolyte systems, including my heart. As a result, I felt weak, my memory was poor, I kept dozing off, and experienced muscle cramps. I often almost passed out on my way to university.

People kept commenting on my weight loss, thinking it was to do with some part-time modelling I was doing, but no one asked the right question. *What is making you not eat?*

My first binge was right after the earthquake and tsunami, which happened in Japan in 2011. I was 20 years old. I was deeply saddened to see so much loss for a country I loved. I was feeling stressed, looking after my grandfather, who was suffering from dementia. I felt isolated, and worst of all, my university boyfriend who I really counted on and could turn to for support let me down. I called him on Skype.

'Hey, so I need to talk to you,' I said, smiling bravely. I was in desperate need to release the tightness in my chest. But when I looked into his eyes, they were sad and teary. He looked away from the screen, and it was clear there was something he was trying to hide.

'Let me go first,' he butted in. Before I could continue, he began to tremble, and his voice began to break as he told me he had been seeing another girl. I felt the colour draining from my face. I hung up the call, unable to cope. Everything deleted like the past two years were gone.

He was my first serious relationship and first love. I never thought him capable of breaking my trust. I had to let him go, knowing it would hurt for some time. But nothing heals the past like time.

I was in a very dark headspace, feeling like I had no one to talk to.

It may come as a surprise, but eating disorders are also considered mental health conditions.

Mine involved extreme restrictions of food intake and then eating large amounts of food in a single sitting.

Regardless of the type of eating disorder, the common result among all eating disorders is they cause serious physical, physiological, or social impairments.

THIS GIRL CAN (SOMETIMES)

People often think of stunning slim models when they think of eating disorders, but this is not the only way that someone with an eating disorder will look. Not everyone who has an eating disorder is really thin, just as not everyone who is thin has an eating disorder.

After two months of starving myself, that night, something snapped. Lying in bed, my eyes snapped open. After avoiding eating food for so long, I hurried down the stairs to the fridge and cleared it out. The fridge began beeping as I had it open for too long. I closed it and reopened it again, the glow illuminating my crazed eyes. My first binge lasted an hour. I ate everything and anything. I was in emotional and physical pain. Leftover cold foods and even frozen foods. Any tinned goods were demolished. Catching my reflection in the glass cabinet, I looked like a wild beast, fingers covered with a mix of sticky rice and sugar. A powerful headache surged from consuming so much food; my body was reacting to the masses of sugar in my blood system. On the wooden floors, 2am, I curled up into a ball wanting to die there and then.

The next day, I went to college as usual. Avoiding my friends, I kept my head down in classes. I came back home and ran up the stairs, closing the bedroom door without even greeting my ojiichan. This breaks my heart still today. He was unsure what was happening and didn't know how to help. I cried into my pillow, until, exhausted, I fell asleep. It wasn't long though until my eyes would snapp open in the middle of the night and I would run downstairs to scour the pantry, looking for something to stuff my face with and numb my pain yet again.

The binges kept happening, and I would phone home crying without really explaining what was happening. It got so bad, mum booked the soonest flight she could to come to Japan.

When she saw me, I was 47kg. Healthy for me is around 70kg. She couldn't recognise me. She started making my meals, ensuring they were all balanced with nutrition. I could taste the love she put into preparing my food. She helped me with my studies and looked after my ojiichan.

During the nights, she tied herself to me so when I would wake up in the night and get up to eat, it would tug on her foot and wake her up, too. This worked on the first night, but the second night I carefully undid the knot and slipped downstairs. There was like a switch in my brain that wanted food, and there was no stopping me from getting it.

Although mum wished me to go back to England to get help, I insisted on finishing university not wanting to drop out, so she helped me stay committed. What I didn't realise, being trapped in my vicious eating cycle, was that mum was stressed just as well and had lost weight. It was because of her positivity, her light and love that I got through university. Her resilience and strength was, and still is, breath-taking.

For being selfish and not seeing my mum's pain, I forgive myself, here and now.

As soon as I was back in England, I saw an eating disorder specialist. She was expensive, and her counselling felt impersonal. Driving up, the sky was moody, a lone oak tree stood by itself on the hill.

Grace was elderly and wore bright pink lipstick, her hair dyed silver. Fingers covered in chunky jewellery. Behaving like a cool aunt, she stated how I looked healthy and normal, chatting to me as if we were friends and she knew me.

I didn't feel healthy. I especially didn't feel normal.

I told her how I'd been clearing the cupboards, eating raw cake mix and feeling numb. I looked at her and saw it. I saw judgement in her eyes.

'Why didn't you cook the cake mix?'

'I wanted to eat it quickly…I don't have much control…'

THIS GIRL CAN (SOMETIMES)

'Well, that's no good, is it?' I hung my head in shame.

I left feeling ashamed and low. Building a rapport, a healthy relationship, is the foundation for any work to be done with a counsellor. I didn't know then, but judgement and shame were feelings a counsellor should never inflict.

If a client is feeling numb, and you sense maybe suicidal, it is essential to explore and see if there are feelings of ending one's life. It can be incredibly difficult to ask, but when I met Dr Jean Rias and she asked me, 'Are you feeling suicidal?' and I had the space to respond with, 'Yes,' it felt as if a foot had been lifted from my chest. I could breathe, I could talk about it, and there was no judgement or shame.

Grace said I could call anytime, yet when I called her having uncurled myself from a suicidal ball, a real time of need, she didn't pick up and never returned my desperate voicemail. I felt betrayed and alone. To say something and not follow through is absolute poison for a counselling relationship.

Fortunately, my family supported me. All items which contained sugar were thrown out or hidden. It was a challenging summer, and my dad and brother didn't quite understand what I was going through.

I had once discovered a secret stash of food which led to a binge, clearing out the kitchen. My brother came home to find me howling on the floor, surrounded by empty food packages and the kitchen a mess. After witnessing this, he developed an empathy he didn't have prior.

When I went back to university in London, my roommate had a lock for her cupboard and fridge so I couldn't access her food which could trigger a binge. But it still didn't stop me. I had become addicted to sugar, and when the brain switch flipped, I was on a mission nobody could stop.

For those of you who don't know how sugar and the brain work, here is a basic and brief summary:

When you consume sugar, it triggers the release of dopamine chemicals in a part of the brain associated with reward and pleasure. If you're addicted to sugar, a spike in dopamine levels represents the anticipation of reward, rather than the actual reward (from eating sugar) itself. But the effects are blunted when you eat sugar because the brain is over flooded with dopamine neurotransmitters at the thought of consuming it.

Addiction is a compulsion to trigger pleasurable sensations in the brain, and the thought of consuming sugar could stimulate the release of dopamine in the reward centre of the brain. I was addicted to this pleasure release, so I would scramble my hand in the small gap around the locked cupboard door and tug on anything which could be pulled out. Crisp packet. Success.

Refined sugar foods act on the reward centre of the brain and have a short-term impact on mood. After consuming the food - interesting to note sugar affects the same parts of the brain as heroin and cocaine - I would come crashing down.

When I attempted to quit eating sugar, I experienced withdrawal symptoms, which caused an imbalance in the brain as it adjusted to perform with high levels of dopamine.

Dopamine provided me with temporary feelings of happiness, pleasure, euphoria and satisfaction. But it was influencing my memory and brain learning.

It was a challenging addiction.

When I ate refined sugar, such as white bread, crisps, chocolate, etc., my body and brain craved more sugar; my blood sugar level spiked as dopamine was released in the brain; hunger and cravings set in, reinforcing the need to eat more sugary food; and blood sugar levels fell. This led my body to crave another 'sugar high' to increase blood sugar levels and induce the feeling of pleasure. This cycle of addiction explains how difficult it is to give up sugar and the grasp it had on my life.

Furthermore, my period had stopped completely for a year. I became concerned about the damage I had caused to my body, and if I would be able to have children in the future.

During my states of undernourishment in Japan, my body didn't have enough 'fuel' to run properly. This meant my body needed to prioritise which were the most important bodily functions. Processes that are not essential to staying alive, such as growth and reproductive function, may get less energy. The functionality of the hypothalamus, the control centre in your brain which regulates many of the hormonal fluctuations within the body, can become suppressed, and normal hormonal fluctuations like those that regulate the menstrual cycle may be altered or, in my case, halted.

After some time, my eating was becoming more manageable. I could have one meal and not binge on two more. I decided to remove refined sugars completely from my diet, so the temptation was not there. But mental illness is never this simple. I started shoplifting.

Now, this is not uncommon, I learnt, reading up about it after I first stole a bottle of wine - one addiction replacing another. Binge eating is an addictive behaviour, in the same way drug users experience intense pleasure. It is the memory traces set down on the neurons in the pleasure parts of the brain that make it so difficult for the binge eater and drug abuser to stop the activity.

My shoplifting was becoming a frequent occurrence, and eventually, I got caught. I had taken some crackers at a health store, and the police were called in. They were very confused, seeing me in my work attire and Prada handbag. I explained my situation: that I had no control and it was an impulse, and I was seeking professional help. I wrote down my doctor's details for them. Fortunately, it did not go on my record. One of the officer's had a Japanese wife, and when I explained my turbulent time in Japan during the earthquake and tsunami, he seemed to take pity on me. The shoplifting and the self-hatred and depression become good motivating factors for me to seek help and learn how to end this cycle.

After that shoplifting incident, I would call my mum entering any shop, listing each item I put in the basket.

It has also been my experience that all of these impulsive activities ended when I gained control over the way I eat and do my shopping. The better enabled I was to fight the impulse to binge and shop, the less frequently I would engage in the binging and shoplifting. Gradually, my need to binge and shoplift decreased, bringing with it increased self-esteem and decreased depression.

The help and support of a therapist and nutritionist, both trained in eating disorders, is an excellent way to get this condition under control. It was just unfortunate I did not feel supported by my eating specialist.

I am now very aware and mindful of what I eat. If I have too much sugar, then still, even after eight years, it can give me a headache or a desire to eat more food. Now that I am aware of this, I can cope better.

CHAPTER 36

*I intend to accept my body today, love my body
tomorrow and value my body always*

Dear Eating Disorder

*You are always there. Sometimes I don't notice you, but you
have this way of reminding me when you feel you've been
ignored.*

*I try to talk back to you when you urge me to overeat or
when you discipline me not to eat, but you fuel me with
anxiety.*

*Our relationship is overwhelming. This may be hard to
hear, but I sometimes feel fearful of you. I'm always left
exhausted after talking with you. This letter is my effort to heal
and understand.*

*You have shown yourself as binge eating, you have shown
yourself as purging, you have shown yourself as an obsession
with exercise and weight, but you are more than that.*

*Sometimes, you are the voice behind my actions. The terror
of eating a cinnamon bun came from you. I don't understand
why you need to be so controlling, how you can be so cruel,
not only to my physical body but to my personality.*

*You are the longest relationship I have been in. But why do
we never celebrate? You devour joy - it seems to keep you alive.*

It has been easier to keep you a secret from those closest to me, and maybe this was hard for you. But let me explain. The more I let others in on my relationship with you, the more I fear you. You have trapped and isolated me from other connections and people. I feared my confident reputation being pierced by you. For every feeling of pain and suffering and insecurity that you have numbed, you have numbed a moment of true joy and close connection. Relationships have failed because of you, you have cost me letting others in because I felt I didn't have a choice.

You suffocated me, you didn't give me the space to live and breathe.

I hate the way that you have stolen precious moments of joy and fun and celebration at dinner with friends, managing your constant anxiety about losing control of me if I drink, if I eat the dessert, if I get the pizza and beer instead of the salad.

Did you know I no longer trusted myself, fearing the binges and purges that I am capable of, fearing the voice of my own hunger? You stole my trust.

I'm tired of your promises. I realise now you promised a forgiveness and identity that is not yours to provide.

I'm sorry that you felt I could never measure up to your standards. I should have eaten less, ran more, and trained in the gym longer.

I have outgrown your thinking, the universe is infinite, and so is my ability to create, live and love.

Please understand. You wreaked chaos on my physical body. I felt confused about when I was hungry and when I was full. I could no longer trust myself to know what my body needed.

In Japan, I felt my body slowing down, deteriorating and exhausted by the mental battle, the physical implications, and the emotional confusion.

You thought you were helping me in my time of need, as a way to survive, but that has passed now, it is time for me to explore a more loving and healthy relationship.

Please don't say I haven't tried. I have embraced you with love, but you push me away time and time again. My worth and my value take a deep plunge when you start your rampage of hate against me.

I have had enough. You have served your purpose. Thank you, but it is time for us to heal and move forward.

I no longer wish to feel numb, I no longer wish to avoid. I am ready to be present for my life.

The pain and the unknown are a part of the journey, and I want to experience it from now on.

I am enough.

With love. X

THIS GIRL CAN (SOMETIMES)

CHAPTER 37

Identity - right about now I'm 50/50

When living in Japan during my year abroad at Waseda, I had an identity crisis. I would specifically be feeling confused about who I was ethno-culturally. I would often ask myself, 'Who am I?' And I didn't know the answer.

My visits in Japan had always been for only two weeks, so I never felt the need to submerge myself. But whilst living there, I was determined to become fluent, establish work connections and build Japanese friendships. What happened in the end, is spending too much time immersing myself in Japanese society left me lonely and confused about who I really am.

I have Japanese blood, therefore the feeling of acceptance should have come easily to me.

What I soon realised was that Japanese society tends to respect groups rather than individuals. Japan seemed intent on always showing their best face and being concerned about how other people saw them rather than how they saw themselves.

This outlook was not healthy for me. I found myself beginning to care too much about what others thought of me.

The Japanese seem to me like group-oriented people who are required to act as a group most of the time, trying not to stand out from other members of the group. This is not a matter of good or bad. It just seems to be a fact of life that the strictly adhered to unspoken rules help harmonise their society, and not following them might result in negative consequences.

I experienced this in outings with my Japanese family and Japanese friends.

I once had a small rip in my tights, and my Japanese friend said, 'You need to change quickly.'

'Why?'

'Because it's embarrassing!' he exclaimed in disbelief.

I took them off in the bathroom, and he nodded when I came out as if to say, 'That's better.' Relief washed over me as I found myself needing his approval that I looked okay.

This would have never happened in the UK. A small rip would go unnoticed, people are welcome to dress in their own style. But to do this in Japan meant you stood out, and I didn't want to stand out.

Appearance seemed to be very important in Japan. Perfect makeup and hair. Living there, I felt scruffy and obviously foreign. I felt big in comparison to my slim cousins and friends. My aunt, on multiple occasions, scolded me on my clothing. I had to go back inside to wear leggings under a dress I considered one of my longer dresses. It was 30 degrees outside, and the black leggings were not a welcomed addition.

I was concerned my aunt thought of me as a bad influence on my younger cousins because of the way I dressed and how outgoing I was.

As I lost weight, I felt I looked more Japanese and therefore conformed more to the unspoken expectations of Japanese society. I tried to embrace this Japanese side in group situations. Agreeing more and being less opinionated. But this did not sit well with me.

When I worked for Japanese companies and helped out at corporate events for companies such as Honda, I very quickly learned how to play the Japanese role. I smiled, I bowed, and I catered to any and all of everybody's needs around me.

Despite being back in London, the unspoken expectations of Japanese society remained in the Japanese workplaces I found myself in. I was always expected to be the one to make tea for my Japanese male peers, despite being in an HR role of supposedly equal stature to them. I had had enough.

THIS GIRL CAN (SOMETIMES)

CHAPTER 38

Weight

It's amazing how a comment from one person can bring your entire world crashing down. My eyes swell up with tears as I recall this conversation.

Lying in bed, Dice's skin was warm.

'Dice, you radiate so much heat when you sleep,' the tone of my voice light.

'It's because I'm thin, your skin stays cold because you aren't.'

I went silent... 'So, because I'm fat?'

'I didn't say that.'

It seems this conversation and similar misunderstandings happen a lot with Dice and even with others. Any comment regarding my body or weight sends me into a fury of negativity and panic.

At a friend's birthday party - 'You look incredible!' *'But for how long?'* I think, smiling whilst thanking my friend for the compliment.

Buzzing after a World Stages Now performance, I was approached by a lady. Standing with my mother, she said gesturing at my mum, 'How come you are so thin...' then looking at me '...and you're... not...' She looked confused, not sure if mum and I were really related.

Little did she know, I've struggled with body image since college. Furthermore, it felt triggering to my experiences in Japan.

My heart sank, and I was silent on the drive home. Tears streaming down my face, mum reassured me I wasn't fat, and I'd come such a long way. Lexi reassured me how strong and amazing my body is and how much it does for me every day.

I felt their love. But the damage was done. I hadn't been feeling confident in my body the past few weeks. I thought about purging or going for a long run once I got home.

Instead, I took a long hard look at myself in the mirror unclothed. Seeing the marks on my stomach where my jeans had been fastened, I broke down crying and climbed into bed.

At that moment, I decided today would be the day I start my blog. Something positive will come from this. A safe space to share my thoughts and feelings and, hopefully, I can help others in some way. Words can carry so much importance and meaning. They have the ability to make someone's day, or in my case, on that occasion, break someone's day.

I have worked hard on liking my body. Before I moved to London and met Jake, there was a year where I was so overweight I did not get out of bed for three months. I was experiencing depression without realising it. I wasn't suicidal, but I was very unhappy.

The Sean T Insanity commercial would be on every morning as I lay sad in bed, and after the 50th time watching it, a sudden determination to get fit struck again. My mum bought the DVDs for me. She would sometimes watch or do Tanya's moves. Tanya always provided the exercise modifications by Shaun T's side. Mum never failed to encourage me before and after each workout. My one regret was not taking the before and after pictures to show my body transformation and weight loss, to receive the free Insanity T-shirt which was offered as an incentive to complete the two-month program.

It wasn't easy. The first session, I gave up halfway through because it was hard and I was very heavy. I felt pretty useless, and I left it for two days before coming back to it with new determination. Two months later, I completed it. The hardest workout of my life. This is how I know I can get through anything. If I could drop 10kg through the Insanity program, I knew I could carry on and do harder things.

My body is incredible. It can run, it lifts, it flows, it is strong. So why do I pinch at my stomach and criticise it in the mirror? Most Western women struggle with their body or appearance at some point in their life. This pressure we may have felt at some stage or another to have the perfect body, to look a certain way, needs to change. Something stuck with me for a while after my relationship with Jake. He made the comment once that I looked better with makeup on and I needed to lose weight. Screw him. I look great with or without makeup, and my body is my own and not his to pass judgement on.

This is a constant daily journey, and there are days where I struggle with my body, weight, and its appearance.

To my Beautiful Body,

You are beautiful. You fill me without the fear of having to take up more space. Space that sometimes I feel unworthy to occupy.

You promise to always be there whenever I need you

With much love. X

THIS GIRL CAN (SOMETIMES)

CHAPTER 39

Will this make me gain weight?

I was sat with Lexi on a bench by one of our favourite coffee places. She had bought a cinnamon bun, and so had I. I had been doing a two-month detox, determined to lose some weight and tone up. Holding the moist cinnamon bun in my hand, my breathing became shallow, my palms starting to sweat as fear gripped me. Thoughts started running wild in my head.

'Will this undo all my hard work?' I thought to myself. 'It is just a bun...eat it, treat yourself.' I then panicked. 'But will this trigger a binge?' My inner self responded with, 'You are with Lexi, this is a safe person to eat this with...' and so would go on the never-ending internal debate.

Developing an anxiety around eating sweets or foods classed as unhealthy often happens to me. Second, third-guessing every decision I make can be tiresome. Lexi clocked the long silence. I was now on the edge of tears, brain stressed, which led me to blurt out loud, 'This cinnamon bun is stressing me out!' Lexi, slightly surprised by the sudden outburst, said 'Okay, let's break it down.' And so we did.

I have a constant battle in my mind when it comes to sweet or indulging foods. I calculate if I deserve it, have I worked out to counter the calories, how will I feel after...etc. One time when Dice wanted fish and chips, I had a ten minute meltdown in the car, deciding if I wanted to eat fish and chips. This is a meal I consider unhealthy, and overeating has always been a problem for me. I didn't want to feel obliged to work it off over the following days.

I decided sharing the cinnamon bun was the way forward. I realise, similar to me, there must be many girls who experience these anxieties and feelings before and after consuming food.

After completing my two-month detox, I could fit into my dresses, and it felt amazing. But then the fear creeps in. 'How long can I keep this body shape for; is the feeling only fleeting, etc.'

My fear was correct.

It wasn't maintainable. After returning to normal portion sizes and having the occasional pizza or beer, I tried on the dresses a couple of weeks later. Unable to do the zip up, I collapsed onto the bed disgusted with myself. All that hard work for nothing. Spending the evening crying, I came to the realisation I was left with the choice to either diet and lose the weight again, or accept I am now this body size and I am able to indulge occasionally and eat bigger portions with this new body size. A moment of clarity embraced me. I came to the decision to accept my body as it is now. I train, I lift weights, and I can run and I cook healthy meals, so there should be no shame in having a beer and pizza on a Saturday night.

Everybody's body is different. Healthy and normal on me will look different on you. I wish to dismiss diet culture, weight loss supplements and a health care system which can sometimes deceive young or vulnerable minds into thinking they don't fit into the standard healthy society. Let me stress again. Healthy can look different to anyone. One of my favourite influencers has the hashtag #normalisenormalbodies. YES. Always speak your truth. The world needs a new normal, which is not the unattainable body.

I ask myself now what would I like to eat? How do I want to feel during eating and after eating? I would like a pizza and a beer and my intention is to be relaxed whilst enjoying the pizza and beer. I now try to welcome the feelings of guilt, the questions. *Can I justify having this? Did I go for a run this morning?* I allow these feelings to emerge, acknowledge them, and accept it's okay to feel food guilt. I try my best to let those feelings be light, and as long as I'm mindful when I eat and have feelings of contentment post-eating, I can have that pizza and beer.

Healing one's body image is a long and complex process, and accepting you don't need to put your life on pause because you aren't happy with your body and feeling unworthy needs shaping into a new reality. Whatever stage your body is at, try to accept and love it. It really does amazing things for you.

THIS GIRL CAN (SOMETIMES)

CHAPTER 40

Shop until you drop

Palms sweaty, my finger hovers over the purchase button on my phone. Heart thudding, I know I don't need this swimsuit, I mean, I already have eight different pairs of swimwear, but it's late, and the rational part of my brain is getting firmly ignored. I click purchase. The adrenaline rush, the sharp inhale, brain lit up. But then the guilt creeps in...

Sometimes my spending can be out of control, and that's where I have Dice and mum to keep me grounded with my money as I know I can be reckless with it. More often than not, it's not about the money. It's about the feeling of being out of control. I'm tempted by the excitement impulse brings, the rush, the experience of feeling unstoppable, and I purposely provide no space to stop and think about what I'm spending my money on.

I have read horror stories about people with bipolar racking up tens of thousands of pounds of bills after experiencing a period of mania, taking years to pay back the debt and needing to borrow money from family and friends - the guilt and shame they experience crippling them.

To prevent this from happening to me, I put safeguards around managing my money when I'm feeling well. This is to protect myself when feeling too low to organise myself or too high to care. I've always found banks and creditors very helpful when I tell them that I have bipolar and ask them to provide extra safeguarding.

Furthermore, with my current counsellor, we have discovered that my online shopping occurs in the evening when I am unable to sleep and feeling low. I now leave my phone in another room and use an Alexa (Echo Dot) as my alarm and have my audiobooks read aloud by Alexa before I sleep. This has proven very helpful.

This is all part of my ongoing struggle, managing impulses and the urges to shop.

Taming the binge disorder was tough. Managing the bipolar and shopping addiction is tough. But it has made me resilient, and I believe I have the strength to overcome any hardships that come my way.

CHAPTER 41

It's already yours

Manifestation has become one of my key recovery tools for my mental health.

Whilst reading *The Secret* by Rhonda Byrne, I began to reflect on my experience of manifestation. The overall message in *The Secret* is everyone has the ability to create their own reality. In other words, thoughts can become things.

I wish to discuss this because this is something everyone has access to and can help with any part of your journey.

When I was 8 years old, my family would read *The Sunday Times*, and in the back would be *The Funday Times*, this section for children. Each month, there would be a drawing competition. Sitting cross-legged in my bedroom, I remember vividly saying to myself, 'I will win this competition.' Confident child, I know, but I knew what I needed to draw to win this competition. In *The Funday Times* was a variety of cartoon characters; I needed to pick out six of the favourites, have them sit on the couch and style it like the characters in the TV show, *Friends*. After drawing it, I asked for a stamp from my mum.

'What do you have there?'

'Ah, wait and see,' I smiled. As a child, and even now, I would keep the processes and dreams to myself, action it and then share the results. I think this stems from me not wanting anyone to dismiss my dreams or doubt me.

I walked to the post box around the corner from me and with the envelope in both hands, posted it, saying, 'I will win this competition.' All my thoughts the following days were of winning the prize and seeing the reaction of my parents.

A week later, I received a letter saying I had won the competition.

A more recent example: at a yoga festival I was teaching at, there was a stall selling beautiful yoga mats. However, I couldn't justify spending £40 on a mat I didn't need. Instead, I purchased a beautiful bespoke necklace with a Hand of Fatima pendant. The lady went on to tell me there was a competition where if you posted a picture on social media with any of the jewellery bought today, there was a chance to win one of her lovely yoga mats. In that moment, I had my heart set on winning the yoga mat. That week I visualised winning the mat and planned my outfit and backdrop carefully to have the best picture highlighting the jewellery. When the competition deadline ended, I was announced the winner.

Now this could be thought of as luck, or maybe not many people entered the competition, but I believe I manifested this to happen.

This outlook changed how I saw my world. When I'm feeling good, I emit a powerful frequency that attracts good things which will make me feel good. During these times, I pounce on my laptop with enthusiasm and begin writing. I have the power to change anything because I am the one who chooses my thoughts, and I am the one who feels my feelings.

If you surround your thoughts with what you want and positive energy, there will be a positive outcome.

CHAPTER 42

Listen as your day unfolds, challenge what the future holds, try and keep your head up to the sky, lovers, they may cause you tears, go ahead, release your fears. Herald what your mother said, read the books your father read, try to solve the puzzles in your own sweet time...

It's half past one in the morning. I couldn't sleep, so I fired up my laptop and started tapping at the keyboard. Dice and I often do long-distance in our relationship, and since Dice has been staying with me, sleep and I have been best friends. But, during this particular night, I had woken up abruptly, feeling panicked.

Yikes. I'm turning 30 in seven days.

I found the list I had written when I was 18. Things to achieve before 30:

1. To be self-employed
2. To publish a book
3. A reputation for being exceptional at my job
4. My own flat and independence
5. Friendships filled with tummy-aching laughter
6. Someone to dream big with

THIS GIRL CAN (SOMETIMES)

Congratulations to me. I have ticked each of these off, yet I still feel uneasy.

My main concerns are now: am I adulting well? Do I have my shit together? Is my mental health in check?

I have never understood why we as humans have been conditioned to think that there's nothing scarier than turning 30. Women are conditioned to fear age and our reflection in the mirror if it doesn't match the societal expectation. It should be fine if a woman never wants to have a ring, a baby, or a husband…and although these aren't key factors of success for me, they were/are for some of my peers. In Japan, you are considered a 'Christmas cake' – past your sell-by date - if you aren't married by 30. In the UK, I feel it is frowned upon if you have no savings and are still living at home with your parents.

Turning to my dear friend, Google, I typed in '*anxiety over turning 30*', and soon came to the conclusion that most of the articles and lists out there are UTTER GARBAGE. Some actually fuelled my anxiety. I understand we can view our twenties like the 'golden years', replaying the best bits on a loop sometimes, forgetting that we spent some of that time broke, heartbroken, and with no idea what we wanted to get out of life…But with this particular list on thirty great things about turning thirty, I had many concerns:

1. **You will have financial security** - I DID NOT spend my 20s climbing the career ladder, therefore in my 30s I am not on the type of wage where I have some disposable cash to enjoy myself.
15. **You can travel the world** - Who made this list? With what money?
17. **Acne goes away** - LIES. I have the biggest spot on my chin right now, ready to explode.

THIS GIRL CAN (SOMETIMES)

20. **No more school, dissertations or essays** - I'm back in education, so essays are still a must.
25. **You'll likely be in the prime of your looks** - Is this writer saying my looks will deteriorate from now? Is it all downhill from here? I was quite happy thinking I would age like fine wine.
30. **You worry less about small things** - I definitely still sweat the small things. Did that message sound too clingy? Does Dice think I'm a good human?

It's worrying that lists like this exist. I found the funny side to it, but for someone else, this list could be really disheartening. I hope in this chapter to explore some of my concerns and what turning 30 feels like for me.

Upon reflection, turning 30 for some reason feels like a huge milestone in my mental health journey, and I think it's because I survived the rough times in my 20s, and that is quite the achievement in itself. However, turning 30 will not give me this amazing newfound sense of confidence that all articles seem to mention.

With every year, I do feel I know myself better and feel more full as a human. In the past three years, I have done so much growing. I feel Lymington was a safe place for me to recover post-breakdown, but now my broken wings have healed. I would like to soar and explore more outside this bubble.

Not only have I physically outgrown clothes, accepting and loving my fuller body, I have also outgrown friendships. This has been hard to navigate, but energies shift, priorities change, and that's okay. Letting go of past relationships has been important. I try not to spend so much energy holding on or worrying what other people might be thinking about me.

With the articles not helping me, I searched Netflix to find something numbing, to escape the anxious thoughts regarding turning 30. Instead, I re-watched the documentary, *Feminists, What Were They Thinking?* The second time around, I felt so inspired by these older women in their 50s, 60s and 70s. I was in awe of their strength and courage and the way they spoke their minds. For the first time ever, I felt getting older can be something to look forward to. With my mental health setbacks, I have learnt that more than anything, it is important to appreciate life, as not everyone is lucky enough to experience it.

At 30, you're supposed to be mature and have it together. I still have lemonade in my wine. 30 really is just another number. It's okay that I may be making it up along the way. I can now believe that I'm exactly where I need to be in my life, and progression will come from there.

CHAPTER 43

My mum, my hero, my rock. She gave all her love to me. The greatest gift a human can give to another.

Dear Mum

It's hard to put into words exactly how thankful I am for you and everything you've ever done for me. My upbringing and life with you and dad has shaped me. There's never been a time I couldn't count on you both.

You're my support system, my rock and my life. You believe in me and praise me in my darkest moments. You cheer me on and push me even when I want to give up.

You are the reason I am who I am today.

When I competed in my first competitive sailing event, and I didn't want to sail anymore after, you were loving and kind. 'That's okay, if you don't enjoy it, we can try something else.'

It is because of you I am strong, loved and supported. I take chances and live because I know you and dad are behind me every step of the way. It is because of you and dad, I will continue to flourish in life.

Thank you for everything you've ever done for me and ever taught me. Thank you for teaching me to care and to have a giving heart. Thank you for teaching me to laugh, because laughter is worth more than gold. Thank you for my work ethic, teaching me to work hard in life, because it will pay off.

Thank you for teaching me that it's okay to fail, to fall and cry, because there's always another chance.

After all, it's the failures and mistakes that teach us in life.

Thank you for being my biggest support, cheerleader, and always believing in me. Thank you for always being a phone call away, whatever the time zone.

The moments I don't want to be on this earth, it is your love which always stops me from acting on any impulses.

Thank you for helping me fly on my own. Thank you for teaching me how to love unconditionally, and most of all, thank you for loving me unconditionally no matter what.

Love

Your one and only daughter.

CHAPTER 44

"Fully grieve your losses and also let yourself feel the full weight of your joys" - Morgan Harper

Every time I had a breakup, my mum would come up to London with our dog Luffy, to help me get through the difficult times. My hope is one day to buy her her dream car. This is the least of what she deserves.

My father has taught me what kindness is. My brother has taught me what being hardworking and being humble looks like. My Auntie Jacque and Uncle Merv have always showered me with praise and support.

I can always talk to one of them when I'm struggling. If I can't talk to my family. Dice, Fli or Lexi are always a message away. They have gotten me through some dark times and are always the first to remind me I can do the hard things, such as sitting with my thoughts.

I have learned that we can't simply switch ourselves on and off as we choose, despite the number of times I had wished for the magical off-button or pill.

As humans, we need time to withdraw, shed our tough armour, and be vulnerable. When this happens, something magical occurs - an alignment in chakras, or a hum of energy, just allowing yourself the space to be sad and love yourself regardless.

If you can't talk to a family member, talk to your GP, Google what communities are out there or call/see someone within the many mental health services available.

You can't stay in the storm forever. Trust me.

Since my breakdown, I have the future dream to help people with mental health issues. I never would have taken this career path if it wasn't for my own experience with mental illness.

SO, TO CONCLUDE

Living with bipolar teaches you a lot about yourself, about mental health services, about medication…and sadly often about stigma, shame and discrimination.

Not everyone with a diagnosis of bipolar disorder experiences psychosis, but I did. It's more common during manic episodes. But just to be clear, it can happen during depressive episodes, too. If you're feeling depressed, wanting to self-harm or kill yourself, first of all, talk to someone. If it can't be a friend or family member, contact your GP, care co-ordinator or local mental health crisis team as soon as possible. Just reach out. I know this can be incredibly difficult to do and just saying out loud, 'I'm feeling suicidal,' is tough, but trust that sharing how you are feeling is the beginning of your journey.

Everything starts with accepting, acknowledging and loving yourself. Love yourself enough to take your dreams seriously. Acknowledge the power of your thoughts and feelings. Accept whatever stage you are at in your journey.

MY CLOSING THOUGHT

Never underestimate the importance of a difficult life experience. There is always an opportunity to learn something new about yourself and grow as an individual.

It's taken me a while to share my story. I have discovered that there is so much more to life, and I see the light. The love I receive is blinding and I have doses daily from amazing family, friends and clients who never stopped believing in me, even when I couldn't believe in myself. I trust my career and the path I am on. I am resilient, and I will continue to dream and share. I am now listening. Listening to my mind and body. I will continue to take it slow and embrace the light, which is just as important as embracing the darkness.

Once we are ready to open, changes will happen, and when we change how we perceive life, life also changes. Vulnerability comes from this change, and this is a beautiful, healing necessity.

This girl can! Well, sometimes. And that's okay. It's okay if all I did for that day was survive.

It's Okay

Do you ever look in the mirror

and ask: Is that really me?

Do you ever have days

you want to be a bird,

fly and be free?

Do you ever feel nervous, on edge when alone?

So anxious and frayed

that you can't leave your home?

Has your heart felt so heavy

THIS GIRL CAN (SOMETIMES)

but your mind in full drive?
Have you sat in your car
and silently cried?
On the flip side,
Are there days when no one can bring you down?
You strut not just walk; you swell in your crown.
I just want you to know,
such feelings are all okay
and life goes best when you take it day by day.

Many thanks for reading. I hope you can share your story.

ABOUT THE AUTHOR

Maria 慧 Claridge is half-English, half-Japanese and was born in Lymington, England. She wrote this book with the intention of helping people understand mental health issues.

Printed in Great Britain
by Amazon